BUS

3|24|9 ?

When the Man You Love Won't Take Care of His Health

ALSO BY KEN GOLDBERG, M.D.
How Men Can Live as Long as Women

WHEN THE MAN YOU LOVE WON'T TAKE CARE OF HIS HEALTH

KEN GOLDBERG, M.D.

WITH DAVID SCHOONMAKER

Produced by Alison Brown Cerier Book Development, Inc.

Golden Books
New York

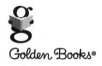

Golden Books®

888 Seventh Avenue
New York, NY 10106

Copyright © 1999 by Kenneth Goldberg, M.D., and Alison Brown Cerier Book Development, Inc.
All rights reserved, including the right of reproduction
in whole or in part in any form.
Golden Books® and colophon
are trademarks of Golden Books Publishing Co., Inc.

Adipex-P is a registered trademark of Gate Pharmaceuticals
Anafranil is a registered trademark of Novartis
Cardura, Viagra, and Zoloft are registered trademarks of Pfizer
Caverject is a registered trademark of Pharmacia and Upjohn
Edex is a registered trademark of Schwarz
Famvir is a registered trademark of SmithKline Beecham
Flomax is a registered trademark of Boehringer Ingelheim
Hytrin is a registered trademark of Abbott
MUSE is a registered trademark of Vivus
Novantrone is a registered trademark of Immunex
Proscar is a registered trademark of Merck
Prozac is a registered trademark of Dista
Redux is a registered trademark of Wyeth-Ayerst
Valtrex, Zantac, and Zoviraz are registered trademarks of Glaxo Wellcome

Foreword by Gail Sheehy copyright © 1999 by G. Merritt Corporation

The Twelve Male Myths about Sex adapted from *The New Male Sexuality* by Bernie Zilbergeld,
Ph.D., Copyright © 1992 by Bernie Zilbergeld. Used by permission of Bantam Books, a division of
Bantam Doubleday Dell Publishing Group, Inc.

The Six Stages of Change (chapter 3) adapted with permission of James Prochaska, University of
Rhode Island

American Urological Association's BPH Symptom Checklist with permission of the American
Urological Association

Partin Tables used with permission of Alan Partin, M.D., Johns Hopkins Hospital

This book is not intended to be a substitute for professional medical advice. The reader should
regularly consult a physician regarding any matter concerning her health or the health of others,
especially in regard to any symptoms that might require diagnosis or medical attention. This book
contains references to actual cases the author has worked on over the years; names and other
identifying characteristics have been changed to protect the privacy of those involved. Medical
science is an ever-changing field; every effort was made to ensure that the medical information
contained in this book was the most accurate and current at the time of publication. Any mention
in this book of actual products does not constitute an endorsement by the publisher or the author
except where noted.

Designed by Suzanne Noli
Manufactured in the United States of America

10 9 8 7 6 5 4 3 2 1

Library of Congress Cataloging-in-Publication Data
Goldberg, Ken (Kenneth A.)
    When the man you love won't take care of his health / Ken
Goldberg, with David Schoonmaker.
       p. cm.
    Includes bibliographical references and index.
    ISBN 1-58238-002-3 (hc : alk. paper)
    1. Men—Health and hygiene. I. Schoonmaker, David. II. Title.
RA777.8.G654 1999
613'.04234—DC21
                                      98-24680
                                         CIP

To the partners of my patients,
with thanks for helping them live longer and better

Contents

Foreword

It has traditionally been assumed that age is kinder to men than to women. My research over the past eight years has revealed a surprising reversal: Today men of age forty and older are having a harder time making a satisfying passage into the second half of their lives than women.

This was the most consistent revelation that came out of interviews with hundreds of men in preparation of my recent book, *Understanding Men's Passages*. Socialized to be eternally strong and to overcome any problem alone, men today are at risk for significant problems with anxiety and depression by the time they reach middle and later life. Some men have to break down—experience a physical blowout or mental plunge into depression—before they can give themselves permission to make a major change in the way they live in order to prolong their lives.

The lengths to which men will go to deny any sign of weakness in their bodies never cease to amaze me. One story I tell in my book depicts the agonizing dilemma faced by the wives of such men.

A Miami man who had built his own successful plumbing business was enthusiastic when his son came home from college and wanted to work with him. But the son, a computer whiz, gradually took over the business. The father was ashamed to admit that databases were foreign to him and backed off. His heart began to feel empty. Anger built up. His breath came hard when he took aerobic walks with his wife and pain laced his chest more and more tightly. He said nothing. A woman in her Flaming Fifties determined to reclaim her figure, his wife believed brisk exercise was good for both of them, and she became impatient. "Why can't you keep up?" He would walk faster.

"Why didn't you tell your wife about your symptoms?" I asked the plumber.

"I didn't want her to think she was living with an old man," he said. "And I don't *feel* old when I walk faster. I just punch through the pain."

One night on their summer camping vacation, the plumber leapt up, stumbled over his wife, ran outside, and threw himself across the hood of his car.

"What are you doing?" his wife shrieked. "Is it your back?"

"My chest."

She tried to talk him into lying on his back on the ground. "I'll call an ambulance."

"No!" he commanded. "I'm going to be fine."

"But you're having a heart attack!"

She ran toward the park ranger's cabin. Her husband outran her and tried to bar her from calling. "Put down the phone! I am *not* having a heart attack!"

He obviously needed help. But at that moment, this proud man felt so overwhelmed by shame, he would have preferred to die than to admit it.

There are real reasons men fear death more than women do. The risk of dying is greater for males than females at every stage of the life cycle. Men age faster than women, get gray hair sooner, lose their sexual drive earlier, rise to anger more quickly, act out their frustration more violently, and may experience the shock of change—such as divorce, down-sizing, death of a peer, departure of the last child—much harder.

Women have a universal cue that they have entered a new stage of life— menopause. What used to be a silent passage, when I wrote a book about it in 1992, is becoming almost as natural a topic of conversation as pregnancy. Women *know* their bodies are changing in middle life. To master that change, they are likely to read books and articles, visit a doctor or a women's health center, ask questions, and start taking care of their health more diligently. Women as they age also form intricate webs of nurturance. Their friendships multiply and deepen. And as the long emergency of motherhood subsides, life opens up for them.

Thus, most healthy women today look forward to middle life with expectations.

Most men look toward middle life with dread.

Why?

They are afraid of losing potency—in all areas of life. But they are even more afraid to admit it. Although men lack the universal cue of menopause, they do go through a middle life slowdown that I have termed MAN*opause*. In 1993, when I first wrote a provocative article about this subject for *Vanity Fair*, I called it "the unspeakable passage." And then, to my delight, a visionary physician spoke up.

* * *

Following the publication of my male menopause article, I had a call from Ken Goldberg, a urologist dedicated to providing men with preventive health care. I learned about his Male Health Institute in Dallas, established in 1988 as the first in the United States to specialize in men's medical concerns. Ken Goldberg is a man's man in the truest sense. He practices urology in a state where the model of the Marlboro Man still holds for many as the idealized image of masculinity (despite the fact that he long ago died of lung cancer). Undaunted, Dr. Goldberg has been a passionate pioneer in the nascent field of men's health.

Men's health? Hasn't the whole medical establishment and pharmaceutical industry been based on the model of men's health and disease? True. Until recently, the National Institutes of Health kept only male rats in their research cages, and drugs were all predicated on male biology. But while the medical establishment uses men's bodies, men themselves abuse them.

I described to Dr. Goldberg how difficult it was to coax men into talking about the physical changes that naturally occur during middle life. He invited me to Dallas to sit in on his men's groups where men who were trying to master MANopause and middle life impotence get together to compare their progress. "I assure you, some of them will talk about your unspeakable passage because they're getting help," said Dr. Goldberg. He was right. These were men forged in the macho Texas tradition. But moving into Second Adulthood without an ethos to replace their performance as young studs, they were as helpless as beached whales.

Bill, for example, had been fishing off the Florida Keys when he hooked a big kingfish. Only 44, he fought his big catch in true Hemingwayesque spirit. Afterward, with his heart leaping like a frog trapped in a jar, he smoked a pack of Marlboros "to calm down." Bill believed he was bulletproof, or better than bulletproof; he didn't need doctors or diets or stress tests. Four days later he was under the surgeon's knife for a quadruple bypass.

It was five years later when I met Bill in Dr. Goldberg's office. He was eager to share with the other men in the group what he was learning about the road back from impotence. The next speaker was a jolly-looking, red-faced man who had put on several bushels full of extra weight in the past couple of years.

"I started in the airline business thirty-five years ago," he told us, "and I stayed in it until June of this year, when I took a nice little early retirement which I was really looking forward to." Almost parenthetically, he added, "I had the cancer last year."

Roy had a prostatectomy, Dr. Goldberg volunteered.

"Yeah. But I've always been in good shape, no problems," Roy insisted.

No problems?

"Well, the sex life changed quite a bit because I'm impotent," he added. "But my friends here at the health center have fixed that up for me." He laughed heartily.

Both men fit the profile sketched by Dr. Goldberg of the typical man in middle life and in denial of his bodily changes. Both men earned over $50,000 a year but were not stimulated by their jobs; they didn't exercise, wouldn't give up smoking, and had gained a dangerous amount of weight. They believed all their problems would be solved when they found a *Playboy* centerfold wife. Each had married younger women and then set about to do everything in their power to please them. At a second session they told what had happened.

In his early fifties Roy began failing to please his attractive, young, second wife. As his erections faltered, his desire flagged. "I wanted to have more sex, but I'd say to myself: *It isn't gonna work tonight, so don't start something you can't finish.*"

"Fear of rejection—is that the worst part?" I asked.

Bill interrupted, "Let me tell you something. When you're lying there at night, and you're trying to make love and it doesn't work, and you hear your wife sigh, like she's saying, 'Not again,' it'll rip your guts out."

Every man in the room leaned forward and hung on Roy's description of the "magic" injection that made him feel like a lion again. The sad part of his story was this: He didn't admit his problem and get help until two years after his young wife had walked out on him.

"Did a wall grow up between the two of you?" I asked Roy.

"I guess so," he said. "To this day I still don't understand why she left."

Married men who haven't been able to perform in the bedroom for years, once they disclose their problem to a doctor, usually reveal the same jarring truth. All the time this eight-hundred-pound gorilla (impotence) has been in their bedroom, *the couple has never talked about it.* Breaking through the silence and shame by admitting they have the problem is the hardest part, say experts. But talking about it, and taking the pressure of performance off the man, can be the most effective medicine of all.

It was a revelation to me to see that when men felt comfortable with a doctor and realized they were not alone in facing a middle life slowdown—and once they learned that the best way to reverse MANopause is to make changes in their diet and do the right kind of exercise, to find their passion, and to expand their network of friends and confidantes—they can make amazing reversals.

In the spring of 1998, when a drug suddenly appeared claiming to counteract impotence, millions of men of age 50 and over came out of hiding and got hold of Viagra any way they could—asking their primary care physicians, begging their druggists, bootlegging it from their bartenders. Everyone was astonished at how many men were suffering from a mid-life sexual slowdown but had remained silent and stoic in their suffering because they didn't know what to do about it.

Apart from making the requisite call to their doctors for a prescription that promises them chemical machismo, however, men still do not go to doctors for routine check-ups. And, when they do go, they don't ask questions. And because most of their doctors are men, the doctors themselves are just as reluctant to ask questions about their male patients' sex lives or to take a history of depression.

Five years ago, Dr. Goldberg tried to talk directly to men by writing an excellent book on men's health, titled *How Men Can Live as Long as Women*. He discovered firsthand how many men are masters of denial. When it comes to their cars, men are fastidious caretakers—getting routine checkups, replacing parts before they burn out, listening for any signs of strain on the motor or coughing in the fuel line. But when it comes to their own bodies, men drive them into the ground. They don't read books about their health. They buy books about money and sports.

To whom does the task fall, then, to take care of a man's health? The save-your-life wife. By default if not by design, it is usually wives who become the caretakers of the aging man's body. So this time Dr. Goldberg is directing his message to women who love and live with men. What follows is a sound, practical, effective guide to maintaining your man's health. Use it well—not in sickness, but in the best of health.

—Gail Sheehy

Preface

In early 1980 my wife, Sharon, our two young sons, and I moved into our first home. After nearly a decade of cramped urban apartments and seventy-two-hour shifts, medical school, internship, and two residencies were finally behind us. Sure, we didn't have enough money to get the place painted, but friends pitched in to put some paint on the walls and linings in the drawers. My family was finally home, and my medical career stood before me. I was a urologist. Frankly, I was excited. I don't remember a time in my life when I wanted to be anything other than a doctor.

I love medicine, and, to be more specific, I love surgery. I'm a scientist at heart, and the precision and skill required to repair the most complicated of all contraptions, the human body, are at once intensely challenging and deeply satisfying. I really enjoy high-tech medicine as well. I was one of the first urologists in Texas to be certified to do shockwave lithotripsy, a noninvasive technique using focused sound energy to break up kidney stones.

After a few years of practicing medicine, though, I realized I was seeing some of the same patients again. I was patching up the same bodies suffering from the same problems. This was certainly good for business, but it began to bother me quite a bit. I began to think that rather than being exciting, there was something senseless about the usual practice of medicine. Why were these men ending up in my examining rooms in the first place, let alone the second time? Why treat them if they would only go out and do the same destructive things again?

At the same time my wife was becoming concerned about my physical condition. While I was establishing a practice, her loving care was helping me give up cigarettes and lose forty pounds through a combination of better diet and exercise. Looking back, I'm a little embarrassed that I represented my other self as a health professional. In those early days my patients certainly didn't find the perfect role model in me. On the other hand, today I can honestly tell any man I see that if I could do it, so can he—especially with the help of a fine woman.

In a very short time my medical practice had an entirely new face. Recalling that the Greek root of the word physician is "educator," I began to look for every opportunity to teach men how to take better care of themselves. No man could escape my offices without a pamphlet explaining one preventive approach or another. Soon I started the Male Health Center, the first medical practice in the country that attempted to attend to all of men's health needs. We also began reaching out to men through corporate health screenings and through the media. What I found, however, still holds true today: It was usually the women, not the men, who were listening.

Women in general are far more enlightened than men about health. Women have different attitudes about well-being and health care—attitudes I'd like to see men acquire. Over the years women who have brought ailing men to me have told me that they care more about his health than his earning power, more about his happiness than his winning ways, more about his soul than his bulging muscles.

After a period of evolution the Male Health Center became the Male Health Institute, a one-stop solution for men's health needs. So far in 1998 we have already done 190 screenings for cardiovascular disease, 245 for stroke, 344 for colon cancer, and 312 for knee problems—all beyond the usual sphere of urology. If I may brag just a little, in the last half of 1997 we were able to attract nearly five hundred teenage males to free health screenings; saw almost three thousand men in the workplace, where they received screenings appropriate to their ages; delivered free screenings to over one thousand men at pharmacies; participated in two clinical trials for impotency drugs; and offered seminars on everything from sexually transmitted diseases to penile prostheses. True, it's only a start, but the signs of acceptance from the men we see are very encouraging.

Men are beginning to listen, and to a large degree it's because women have shown the way. My sincere thanks for the inspiration and insights of many women who have made a difference to men's health: wives, mothers, sisters, daughters, doctors, nurses, physical therapists, social workers, and most of all my wife, Sharon. I'd also like to thank my sons, Jeremy and Josh, who have spent parts of their summers stuffing envelopes; they helped convince me that I was right—some of the time. To the staff at the Male Health Institute and my other offices, thanks for regularly going beyond the call of duty to do what was needed. Many thanks to Dave Schoonmaker who has been, as always, a dedicated and enjoyable collaborator. Thanks also to his wife, Nancy, for adding her insights and to his entire family for their understanding about all those early-morning phone calls. For her excellent word skills and intuitive understanding of what I am trying to accomplish, my thanks go out to Alison Brown Cerier. Gail Sheehy has not only provided the foreword to this book, but also has made numerous contributions to the betterment of male health. Thank you to Bernie Zilbergeld, James Prochaska, Alan Partin, and other doctors and experts who have graciously allowed me to build on their important work. I am also grateful to the many professionals I have cited in this book who are leading the way toward new male attitudes and better health. To the colleagues, too numerous to name, who have checked my words when I have stepped close to the edge of my professional territory, I also owe a debt of gratitude. You have all worked to make men's lives better. Know that you've made a difference and that we're on our way.

In health,

Dr. Ken Goldberg

Part I

"If This Isn't Love"

1

How His Health Affects You

When it comes to their health, most men are living in denial. If the man *you* love was running up the stairs and felt twinges in his chest, would he just shrug them off? Has it been years since he's had a complete checkup? Does he eat a lot of fast food? Does he smoke? Does he have problems with erections? Does he fall asleep in his easy chair many evenings? Does he think that real men tough out their aches and pains?

If many of the answers are yes, he is very typical. Most men fail to follow a healthy lifestyle, to have important tests and examinations, and to identify signs of medical problems. Eventually, they have problems. If your guy's not taking good care of himself, before long he will be a very reluctant visitor to the doctor—or to the funeral home.

Over the years of dealing with men who've let themselves go to a sorry extent, I've come to understand that they aren't the only ones who suffer. Women shoulder most of the burden—from the strains of worry to the hard work of caregiving when men are sick or disabled. Furthermore, many of men's bad health habits (smoking, drunk driving, and others) put women's own health at risk.

In picking up this book, though, you probably weren't thinking about yourself but about him. Put simply: You love him. You want him to be healthy, happy, and headed for a hundred.

Unfortunately, it's not easy to help a man turn around. If you've tried to talk to him about his health, you've probably run up against a stone wall. In this book you'll learn strategies that will get through to him.

Though it may seem he'll stay the same way forever, I've watched many men turn the corner. Men can learn to take better care of themselves. Trust me, I *know* it can happen. With the support and love of a fine woman, I managed to do it myself.

Before we talk about solutions, let's look more closely at his approach to health and its consequences for him and you.

How He Abuses His Health

First, most men don't get themselves to the doctor when they should. Each year men visit the doctor 130 million fewer times than women do (even after adjusting the numbers so that prenatal care doesn't skew the results), and 37 million men haven't seen a doctor in the last two years. Men also go to the dentist less often, steer clear of mental health services, and take fewer medications than women. They are less likely to have their blood pressure checked and their cholesterol tested, even though men under fifty-five are twice as likely as women to have elevated cholesterol levels. Only 60 percent of men at high risk for colorectal and prostate cancer had a digital rectal exam (the simplest early-detection method) in the past year.

How far will a man go to avoid health care? Consider one of my patients, a fifty-six-year-old we'll call Jim. Jim's wife, Sally, an emergency-room nurse, is the only reason he's alive today. One Friday evening Sally noticed that Jim seemed subdued. Later she told me, "He really didn't want to talk much; he'd hardly look up from the TV when I spoke to him. I figured he'd had a rough week and left him in peace. That night he didn't sleep well. He got up to go to the bathroom several times, and tossed and turned. The next day he got positively glum. I asked if there was anything I could get him, and he asked for aspirin. That evening he wouldn't eat dinner. Saturday night was even worse, and by Sunday morning he was clearly in intense pain. I practically had to scream at him to get him to say what was wrong, but finally he told me he hadn't been able to urinate since Friday morning. I put him in the car and drove straight to the emergency room."

Sally called me from there, and I headed for the hospital. Jim was in acute urinary retention from an enlarged prostate, a potentially life-threatening condition. This sort of thing doesn't develop overnight. Jim eventually admitted that he'd been having problems with his prostate for quite some time but "didn't want to bother anyone about it." He'd let it go for so long that the only solution was surgery followed by a catheter. If he'd sought help early, there's a good chance we could have controlled the problem with medication. I could tell you dozens of stories just like this one.

Men not only avoid the doctor's office but neglect basic self-care. Women are far more likely than men to apply sunscreen before they go out in the sun even though they spend less time out there. Furthermore, fewer than half of men check their skin for signs of skin cancer, compared with more than three-quarters of women. Though testicular cancer is the most common solid cancer among young men, nine out of ten college men don't know how to do a self-exam, and fewer than 14 percent do one regularly. Men don't even bother to take vitamins and minerals, despite being more likely than women to eat diets deficient in them.

Most men don't just neglect their bodies, they actively abuse them by what they eat, how they drive, their high-risk sports, their abuse of alcohol and drugs, and even the jobs they take.

You probably see evidence of men's poor dietary habits across the dinner table from you every evening. Men eat far more dietary fat and cholesterol than women do and are less likely to limit red meat. This increases their risk of heart disease and a variety of cancers. They eat less fruit, vegetables, and foods containing dietary fiber, while they take in more salt, sugar, and caffeine. Men are more likely to skip breakfast, the most important meal of the day. These dietary habits can really put on the pounds. Nearly a third of men thirty to forty-four years old—a prime time for the development of future problems—are overweight compared with fewer than a quarter of women.

When they get behind the wheel, many men show disregard for their well-being, not to mention that of others. Speeders and tailgaters are overwhelmingly male, yet three-quarters of drivers observed not wearing seat belts are men. Nearly a third of young men report taking risks while driving "for the fun of it"; fewer than 10 percent of women do. Drunken drivers are almost exclusively male, 96 percent of those apprehended. (Men even like to drink and *walk*: 42 percent of male pedestrians killed by motor vehicles are intoxicated, compared with only 20 percent of females.)

As the statistics on drunk driving attest, the boys have a major attraction to the bottle. Men are five times as likely as women to take more than two drinks per day. Drinking men don't back off to compensate for their impairment; they increase their risk of injury during everything from sports to work to odd jobs around the house. Men are also more likely to abuse illegal substances such as marijuana and cocaine. Three times as many men as women smoke marijuana at least once a week, and twice as many men have tried cocaine. Similar patterns exist for tobacco. Although similar numbers of men and women smoke (28 percent of men, 23 percent of women), nearly twice as many men smoke more than two packs a day. Cigars and oral tobacco are almost exclusively male poisons.

Our sex also has a fascination with risky sports. Skydiving, hang gliding, auto racing, mountain climbing, and contact sports are predominantly male pastimes. Men even add risk to sports that don't have to be risky. We're far more likely than women to swim alone, be intoxicated while swimming (50 percent of male drownings involve alcohol), bicycle at night without appropriate lighting or reflective clothing, and so on. Even in sports pursued more or less equally by men and women, such as skiing and bicycling, men push their limits significantly more often.

A colleague of mine recently told me a story that captures the difference between the ways women and men approach the risky element of sport. He delighted in telling me that a female doctor he knew, already a stunt pilot, had just taken up motorcycling. Obviously, this is one woman who is drawn to high-risk sports. Curious, I asked, "Did she buy a bike and hit the road as a man would?" No, he responded. She had bought the best and most complete protective equipment, taken an intensive motorcycle training course, and ridden the bike almost three hundred miles on an unused runway at her local airport before venturing onto the street among cars. My colleague mused, "Can you imagine a guy taking that much care?"

Men's higher risk of accidents, as well as some other health problems, is related to another bad health habit: lack of sleep. Men sleep less than women—about six hours a night compared with nearly eight hours. Sleep deprivation contributes to 200,000 auto accidents, 3,499 deaths from injury at home, and half of all deaths related to injuries at work (94 percent of which happen to men).

Most people don't go to a doctor for help with sleep problems like insomnia or snoring, but I see a lot of sleep-deprived men because they come to me for help with a major sleep thief: an enlarged prostate gland. The pattern is so common. A forty-something businessman works seventy hours a week, so he doesn't have time to exercise or eat right. Traveling or attending endless meetings, he spends most of his days sitting, his overweight torso centered over his prostate. Come bedtime, he's too stressed out to fall asleep, but a double scotch helps. Within an hour or two, though, he's up for a trip to the bathroom. He'll be up a few more times during the night, too. The only advantage of the pesky prostate is that the discomfort keeps him from dozing off in the boardroom. I'm sympathetic to his desire for a pill that will solve his problem, but I'd rather see him get some exercise, work on his diet, lose some weight, and give up the nightcap—techniques that are likely to work at least as well and to have much better side effects.

Considering how much the average man claims to love sex, it's particularly puzzling that he will put his sex life at risk. A high-fat diet and lack of exercise lead to blocked blood vessels not only in the heart but also in the penis. That's why smoking, heart disease, and impotence often go together. Many men increase their risks of sexually transmitted diseases by having multiple partners. Men are significantly less likely than women to be monogamous. Your man may be utterly faithful to you now, but what about before you became acquainted? Young men begin sexual activity sooner than women and on average have many more partners. Barely a fifth of males remain virgins by age nineteen, and over half of all men have had at least six sexual partners in their lifetime, compared with only a quarter of women. Yet only a third of men who are at high risk of sexually transmitted diseases consistently use condoms.

Finally, men put themselves at risk with violent behavior. Half of American men own guns compared with less than a quarter of all women, and 95 percent of all violent crimes are committed by men. Violence is so much a part of male culture that half of all boys are involved in a fight each year. Three and a half times as many boys as girls consider fighting an appropriate response to someone who cuts in line.

To sum up, men abuse their health by neglecting routine exams and tests, by ignoring symptoms of health problems, by eating the wrong foods, by smoking, and by taking risks with their sports, drinking, sex lives, and violent situations. Of course, the man *you* love may not be guilty of all these charges. He may be better than most in some departments. If so, heap on the praise. There *are* men who work out regularly, watch what they eat, even get their checkups. If you think of him as a man who "won't take care of his health," though, he's falling short in some important ways.

The Toll for Him

When men neglect checkups, eat fast food and thick steaks, drink too much, smoke, and otherwise put their health at risk, they pay a heavy price. The bottom line: Men top women in fourteen out of the fifteen leading causes of death (with the data adjusted to account for women's longer life spans). The death rate for heart disease, the number one killer, is nearly twice as high in men as in women, and men's death rate for all cancers (the number two cause) is one and a half times higher. The statistics for some specific types of cancer look much worse. Lung cancer death rates are twice as high in men, and oral cancers are three times higher. Two out of three people who die from melanoma, the most deadly form of skin cancer, are men. The difference between the male and female approaches to health shows up in changes in the occurrence of colorectal cancer since 1958: a decline of 30 percent in women but only 7 percent in men. I could fill a chapter with similar statistics, but put simply, the death rate among men is roughly twice what it is for women from the time they're fifteen until they hit sixty-four.

Statisticians have known for centuries that women outlive men. Today the difference is six-plus years for whites and nine years for blacks (and fourteen years between white women and black men). Until about ten years ago most of the medical community assumed that something about being male was just plain deadly. It's become increasingly clear that this simply isn't true. So far medical science has failed to turn up a biological smoking gun. Men die early because we behave as we like.

His and Her Chances of Death

At each age, how many men die of the most common causes? How many women? The figures below from the Centers for Disease Control and Prevention are adjusted so that they aren't skewed by women's longevity, which makes them more likely to die from the causes that are related to aging. The adjusted numbers tell the true story.

	NUMBER OF DEATHS PER 100,000 PEOPLE PER YEAR	
CAUSE	MEN	WOMEN
Heart disease	184.9	100.4
Lung cancer	55.3	27.5
Stroke	28.9	24.8
Chronic obstructive lung disease	26.3	17.1
AIDS	26.2	5.2
Motor vehicle injuries	22.7	10.0
Other unintentional injuries	21.4	7.5
Breast cancer*	—	21.0
Suicide	18.6	4.1
Pneumonia and influenza	16.5	10.4
Prostate cancer	15.4	—
Colorectal cancer	15.3	10.6
Homicide	14.7	4.0
Diabetes	14.4	12.4
Liver disease and cirrhosis	11.0	4.6

*Men do get breast cancer, but it is not among the leading causes of death.

The Toll for the Nation

Men's denial of their health affects even national health policy. In 1997 the National Cancer Institute spent about $330 million on breast cancer research and about $60 million on prostate cancer. In the same year about 45,000 women died from breast cancer and about 42,000 men died from prostate cancer. I would never suggest that one source of funding should be robbed for another, but it isn't logical that we spend five times as much money on breast cancer research. The reason for the difference is that women have success-fully lobbied Congress; the men, as usual, have just died quietly. Fortunately, there are signs this is changing. Thanks to intense efforts by a few men, research funding for prostate cancer is expected to be increased for 1998.

The Toll for You

A quick census of the occupants of a Sun City bus will quickly eliminate any doubt that women outlast men. His approach to health may well deprive you of a happy retirement together. Assuming you like having him around, this is the ultimate toll for you.

Long before he leaves you, though, his declining health will be a burden on you. Women are 72 percent of the nonprofessional caregivers of people with chronic diseases. Caregiving can be physically demanding for an aging spouse. And even when the woman takes much of the care on herself, medical expenses can quickly absorb a couple's retirement savings.

A man in poor physical health will probably also have mental problems that will make him unable to contribute fully to a caring relationship. Depression and illness often go together, and physical inactivity makes both worse, especially in older people. Suicide rates hit their peak in men sixty-five and older; if he lives to seventy-five, he'll be almost ten times as likely as you to take his own life. At the very least a man who's working hard to deny his feelings about his health will put emotional distance between himself and everyone else in his life, including you.

Aside from harming the emotional side of a relationship, poor male health can have a devastating effect on the physical relationship. Many women enjoy a sexual peak in their late forties, just when a man's interest and performance may begin to be compromised by poor health habits. A study of Massachusetts men found that one in three men over forty has erection problems. Being overweight and inactive, drinking too much, and smoking all depress libido and, over time, contribute to impotence. In another study, 72 percent of men seeking medical help for potency problems were smokers—and these were the men who bothered to get help. Untreated diabetes (both preventable and usually controllable by lifestyle) almost always leads to loss of erections.

Potency problems cause more than a loss of physical pleasure. Many women consider the penis to be a "love detector." When he doesn't respond, she assumes he doesn't love her or that she has become less attractive. I've seen it so many times: a man whose erections are flagging and a partner whose sense of self-worth is going out the window.

His health habits take other tolls on you, too. If he smokes, your risk of lung cancer and heart disease is greater. If he crashes the car after drinking, you could be in the passenger seat. Sexually transmitted diseases? He's far more likely to bring one home than you are. Some STDs with almost no symptoms can cause you big problems later—including cervical cancer, infertility, and ectopic pregnancy, a life-threatening condition in which an egg is fertilized in a fallopian tube.

Is he participating equally in birth control? Not in most couples. Though vasectomy for men is a safer and less expensive form of permanent birth control than a tubal ligation is for women, many fewer are done each year. The fact that there are more female options for birth control plays a role in who handles the chore, but the simple, economical, and effective condom still plays less of a part in American family planning than it should. And talk about risk-taking: Has he ever wanted to skip the precautions "just this once"?

Also consider the messages he's sending to your offspring. He may pride himself that he can keep up with your son's soccer team despite his pack-a-day habit, but what kind of role model is he when he stands next to the bench with a cigarette in hand? Is it any wonder so many boys grow up thinking that bad health behaviors will hurt the next guy, not them? Even if your husband's attitude toward his health is beyond hope, does he have the right to teach the children his ways?

Clearly he needs to learn that his health isn't his business alone. However, you won't be able to reach him with confrontation or accusations. Let's look deeper into the male psyche to see what *will* reach him.

2

The Bulletproof Male

W hat is it about being male that causes us to imagine we're immune to danger? Do we ignore our health because of our genes or hormones? Or do we *learn* to ignore our health through subtle and not-so-subtle cues from the people around us—messages that society delivers to every man? Social scientists have argued for decades over whether "nature" or "nurture" governs human behavior, but many experts now believe that both play a part. I agree. I also believe that we don't have to live with just the dark side of manhood. Men have inborn characteristics but are quite capable of learning new tricks.

A Caveman in a Suit

The inborn aspects of the male psyche were put there way back in prehistory. Until ten thousand years ago men were hunters. Successful hunters survived, so they were able to pass their genes and their behaviors on to their sons. Unsuccessful hunters didn't survive, and their genes and behaviors died with them. Because evolutionary change takes thousands and thousands of years, adaptations made way back then remain a part of our genetic code today. Inside your man's skull is the brain of a prehistoric hunter.

Consider which male behaviors would have been most rewarded a half-million years ago on the plains of Africa. Hunting is a fundamentally aggressive activity that requires not only certain attitudes about the taking of life but also the ability to set aside concerns about personal risk. Men also had to overwhelm their human enemies. Aggression, killing, and risk-taking became part of the male genetic heritage. Men were also always in competition for the most desirable women. A dominant, aggressive man was more likely to pass along his genes to offspring.

Consider a successful hunter's attitude about his health. If he had a runny nose, would he stay home in the cave and cover up with a fur? If he did, his family would go hungry, and his mate would soon find another man who could do a better job of providing. (In prehistory, as today, a man's wealth—whether in antelope haunches or common shares—is his most seductive characteristic.)

From an evolutionary standpoint, the ten thousand years that have passed since agriculture was developed are a mere moment. Certainly the speed of change in the last two hundred years has totally outrun the pace of natural selection. It will be some time before the characteristics that best ensure survival in the modern world are part of our genetic structure.

Although our inborn characteristics don't always work in our best interest, there is one that can save us: our ingenuity. For hundreds of thousands of years, human ingenuity has overcome the disadvantages of a body that can't run as fast, jump as high, or bring down prey as readily as our animal competitors can. Today, in a world that threatens us in very different ways, we can use that ingenuity to learn to live longer and better lives. Our brains may be best equipped to deal with Stone-Age problems, but we can learn to manage modern ones. After all, men keep our cars running. Why not our bodies?

Lessons in the Locker Room

The self-destructive behaviors rooted in men's brains thousands of years ago are still being reinforced every day. The best place to watch this happen is a locker room. You probably haven't spent much time in men's locker rooms, so let me take you on a tour.

At any place that men work out, the heart of the action is not the weight room or the gym but the locker room. Men's locker rooms—whether at the health club, the country club, or a college athletic center—are social centers where guys work out a pecking order (one that's every bit as important as that in the workplace). As they verbally joust, they exchange clear messages about what's expected of them.

The conversation may drift from professional sports to business to women, but the approach is the same. A successful man makes two points when discussing any topic. First, he demonstrates that he knows more about it than anyone else present—for example, why this or that professional athlete does or doesn't perform at capacity or why so and so (not present) is having marital problems. Second, he asserts that his knowledge places him in a position of authority, not just over the men present but also over those being discussed. If only they would listen to him, their winning performance, profit margin, or connubial bliss would be restored. Of course, there's an implication that he, being a superior example of manhood, doesn't have such problems.

Noticeably missing from every locker room conversation I've ever heard is fallibility. If you could be a fly on the wall while the guys strip off sweaty clothes, you would not hear them discuss their poor investments or their problems with premature ejaculation. The only health topic discussed might be an injury that the person is man enough to play through. Pain can come up in a conversation as long as it's triumphed over or at least ignored. A man may admit that a sickness or injury has caused an inferior performance, but he must not give in to it. He shows up and tries.

Locker room indoctrination starts at an early age. If fathers don't do it, the schools do. The beginning could be the first sports physical, when boys are forced to stand around stripped to their underwear while they're poked and prodded in public. Or it could begin when they have to use a group shower. At a time when boys are feeling insecure about their changing bodies, they're deprived of privacy. The inevitable establishment of the pecking order can be very unkind. Some men never recover from their first sports physical. (There is another way. When my associates and I conduct teen physicals, every boy gets a private room, and the boys are distracted from each other before and after by having professional athletes to talk to, watching videos, and eating healthful snacks.)

When boys, and later men, haze each other in the locker room, the issue is weakness. The interactions attempt to expose weakness, and to succeed, a man must not reveal it.

Since a man's great fear is to expose his weaknesses, it's no wonder he doesn't want to go to the doctor. The doctor might find something wrong with him! When I stand in front of a group of men and tell them that one in three of them has high blood pressure, one in three has an enlarged prostate, one in three has symptoms of prostate cancer, and one in three has high cholesterol, each man is saying to himself, "Not me. It's one of the guys sitting next to me." When neglect of their bodies finally catches up with men, should we be surprised that they refuse to talk about it? They have been taught that to get sick is to be weak. A "real" man ignores his troubles and fights on.

Messages from Parents and Peers

Most people don't realize how young males are when they begin to get the message they should be tough. Studies have shown that most parents treat their daughters and sons differently even when they don't think they do. As infants, boys are less likely than girls to be comforted with a hug or a touch. Physical contact with boys usually involves stimulation—bounces, tickling, and rough play—rather than gentle affection. By the time her son is a year old, the typical mother has already begun to distance herself from him. At a year and a half, boys are left alone to play much more often and for longer than girls. Mothers have been found to worry less about physical injury to their sons than to their daughters. Thus males are encouraged at a very early age to be emotionally and physically distant from others—to be tough.

Parents also talk differently with sons than with daughters. In general, emotions dominate parent-girl conversations, and actions dominate parent-boy conversations. Performance, not compassion, is encouraged in young males. When parents do discuss an emotion with boys, is more likely to be anger than sadness. In fact, an emotion expressed by a boy is more likely to be interpreted as anger than the same emotion expressed by a girl.

Parents and other adults also pass along messages about physical activity and risk. Boys are expected to take part in extended physical play. Fathers are far more likely to wrestle with their sons. Boys are also much more likely to receive physical punishment. They're encouraged to dole it out, too. Three out of four Americans believe that boys *benefit* from a few fistfights as they grow up!

Adults not only encourage stereotypical gender roles but also actively discourage behaviors outside those roles, particularly a male behaving like a female. Since the late 1950s repeated studies have found that boys who cross that barrier—by dress, by modes of play, or even by choosing female playmates—are viewed far more negatively than girls who venture into male territory. Similarly, surveys have shown that parents (especially fathers) are more concerned that their sons exhibit male behavior than that their daughters show traditional female behavior. People expect that sissies will have more trouble later in life than tomboys will.

Once they're in school, boys and girls enforce traditional gender roles even more fiercely than adults do. Both sexes punish those who fail to toe the line. Girls who behave like boys are ignored; boys who cross the boundary are mocked and hit.

As the boy grows up, the entire culture reinforces his gender role. He's rewarded for ignoring pain, taking risks, suppressing emotions, and acting aggressively. A man who does otherwise risks ostracism.

I've seen thousands of men outgrow the behaviors that ruin their health. All too often, though, this happens later in life and only in response to a life-threatening condition. We need to start with boys to help them change before it's too late.

Males and Media

In the movies, the ultimate male is the superhero who puts himself in harm's way to triumph single-handedly over evil. The superhero is physically powerful, takes lots of risks, is immune to danger, and always gets the woman. Tellingly, superheroes are never shown working on their physical prowess. Arnold Schwarzenegger built his gleaming muscles in the weight room, but the characters he plays are never shown working out at the gym. Presumably they got that way because of lucky genes and an iron will.

The media depict sports heroes in similar ways. Every man in America knows who Michael Jordan is, but few have any idea that he has to work to keep his skills sharp. We don't see his predawn workouts, strict diet, and careful attention to medical care. To me the myth that his prowess is God-given only diminishes him. The real hero is the Michael Jordan who works harder than others to make the most of his talent.

Along with male power comes violence, the real staple of most of our entertainment. Men make the biffs, booms, and crashes. Young male TV characters are 60 percent more likely than female characters to succeed through aggression. Adult male characters initiate violence much more often than do women, and they get away with it. Men may take more risks than women do, but they're far luckier. On the daytime soaps the women die off in droves while the men, typically doctors or other authority figures, miraculously escape deadly situations.

In dramas and their commercial interruptions, another province of male characters is boozing. For example, in beer commercials the guys are doing the drinking. The women look on admiringly while the men demonstrate athletic ability and fearlessness. It's no accident, so to speak, that breweries like to sponsor automobile racing. Prime-time TV producers, too, have picked up on men's romance with alcohol. In 60 percent of all evening television programs, at least one character drinks an alcoholic beverage, and two-thirds of them are men.

Cigarette smoking is even more strongly portrayed as a male habit. Among the top money-making movies of the 1980s, men were shown smoking four times more often than were women. Prime-time TV is even worse. Its male stars are six-and-a-half times more likely to light up. As is the case with alcohol, tobacco companies associate themselves with car races and their celebrity drivers. Smokeless tobacco is subtly depicted as a performance-enhancing alternative to smoking for the really athletic man. The Skoal Bandit, indeed.

Sports Illustrated, the magazine most popular among adolescent males, carries more tobacco and alcohol advertising than any other magazine. Beer and cigarettes are being modeled as the male thing to do.

Men at Work

Men also receive messages about physical risk at their workplace. Traditionally, and often still today, men are expected to face personal risk to get the job done and to provide for their families.

For one thing, men are more likely than women to have jobs that are physically dangerous. Although the National Safety Council breaks down worker injuries by male and female, it doesn't even bother for on-the-job deaths; men die on the job so much more often that it's not worth breaking down the statistics. Thankfully, the overall death rate for workers has dropped dramatically over the past eighty years, but a few occupations still pose unusually high risks: mining, agriculture, construction, and transportation. Not surprisingly, most of these jobs are filled by men. There are other ways a man's job can be dangerous, too. An executive who works sixty-hour weeks and endures terrible stress in silence can be killed by his job, too.

Although the military is adjusting (sometimes painfully) its attitudes toward male and female roles, most fighting soldiers are still men. Men in the military deserve our gratitude for risking their lives to defend our country. Still, this is yet another message that a good man is willing to sacrifice his life for others.

Whether on the job or in battle, our culture treats men as if they were dispensable. From the point of propagating the species, they *are.* Our population can flourish with a high ratio of women to men.

I see men every day who have basically accepted that they lack value. Their sense of self-worth has been destroyed, if it ever had a chance to flourish, by relentless pressure from parents, peers, media, jobs, and the culture they live in. Until we can convince them that they *are* worth saving, it will be an uphill battle to save them from themselves. Until they know that their health is important to you and us, it's unlikely that it will be important to them.

3

You Can Make a Difference

Considering that he's had a lifetime of bad lessons about male health, the man you love needs a lot of support if he's to change. If anyone can make the difference, you can, because you know him the best, care about him the most, and are most motivated to keep working until there's success. However, the fact that you do have a relationship rules out some of the most common and effective ways people influence each other. If you were his boss, his sergeant, or the IRS, you could use rewards, flattery, or veiled threats. If you were his mother, you could withhold his allowance.

Nagging doesn't work, either. He'll just tune you out, and you'll only damage your relationship. I suspect that I see the results of nagging far less often than it happens simply because men who are nagged rarely go to the doctor. Nonetheless, I've seen my share of naggers in my office. Men who are nagged usually react in one of two ways: They fight back, or they withdraw. Essentially, however, they're achieving the same goal: to tune out the message. I've listened to a woman badger a man only to have it become obvious that he hadn't heard a word she said. He wasn't listening. Repeating the message more often or more loudly won't work if he won't listen.

So how do you get through to him? First, you have to figure out what kind of help he needs.

The Six Stages of Change

James Prochaska, a professor of psychology at the University of Rhode Island, says that people (both men and women) who change their behavior about health go through six stages. Although Prochaska's techniques are new, they work so well that they are rapidly being adopted by the medical community.

Prochaska says that the person needs a particular kind of support and reinforcement at each of the six stages. Let's see how a woman could help a man at each stage of a common change: stopping smoking.

Prochaska calls the first stage *precontemplation*. The man hasn't even considered changing his behavior. He may recognize that change would be good and may even want to change, but he has no plans to do so. To help a man move beyond this stage, work with him to list the benefits of changing the behavior. He probably knows that smoking increases his risk of lung cancer, but he may not know all the other benefits of stopping. Besides lung cancer the list would include lowered risk of heart disease and stroke; protection from oral, esophageal, and stomach cancer; greatly reduced chance of the incurable lung disease emphysema; reduced likelihood of impotence; more energy; savings of money; sweeter breath; fewer bad colds; and so on. Totaled up, the benefits will look very impressive.

Once a guy breaks through precontemplation, he reaches the *contemplation* stage. He recognizes that the benefits of change are very significant but thinks the barriers are too great. He doesn't think he *can* quit smoking. To break through the contemplation phase, he needs your help to learn how others have succeeded. For a smoker this is a great time to be around former smokers. First of all, they'll tell him that they have quit and that he can, too. At least as important: There's no one more righteously opposed to smoking than someone who has quit.

When a man plans to adopt a more healthful behavior within the next month, he's entered the *preparation* stage. Now he needs your help to make a plan. He will reach a point where he's willing to make a public commitment to the change. He should say to you and to his friends that he *will* quit smoking and make a list of what that entails. Besides the obvious—getting rid of the cigarettes—the ashtrays must go, and it's a good time to clean carpets and draperies to remove familiar tobacco odors. He'll also need to plan how he'll change his habits, which have been wrapped around smoking. If he likes to sit on the porch and have a cigarette first thing in the morning, for example, he might plan to go for a short walk instead.

Stage four is the time for *action*. The cigarettes go out of the house. Even though this step seems the most clear-cut of them all—and it is the most difficult—he shouldn't expect it to be quick. Realistically, the hard work of any change lasts for at least six months, and he needs to be mentally prepared to endure. Prochaska tells his patients to think of this stage as a marathon, not a sprint. Most people who have failed to give up smoking underestimated how long it would take for a change to become a part of their life. The cigarettes may be gone from his front pocket, but they still retain a powerful hold on him. He'll be reminded of them dozens of times a day, and he must be ready to resist the urge to have "just one more."

Once the change is well established, he enters *maintenance*. This is a defensive phase. When he's under stress or emotional distress, he's vulnerable to a relapse. It's important to have plans in place to deal with a relapse when (not if) it happens. What will he do if he's at a party where lots of people are smoking or if he goes through a stressful period at work? During this period the bad habit, established over years and years, is gradually replaced by a more healthful one.

The final stage is called *termination*. When your man reaches this phase, he'll be fully confident that he can handle any situation without resorting to his old behavior.

Although the stages progress neatly from one to the next, in real life the process usually moves forward in fits and starts, and nearly everyone slides back a stage from time to time before moving forward again. When you see your guy slipping, remember what worked at the old stage and help him get moving in the right direction again.

Educate Yourself About Male Health

Before you can help, you first need to learn about male health, which is in many ways different from yours. The coming chapters will make you an authority on what it takes for a man to be healthy. Here's a preview of what you'll learn as you read on.

First we'll talk about actions that can help keep him healthy. You'll learn how to help him get the right medical care, select the right doctor, do regular self-examinations, start exercising, eat better, control his weight, deal with stress, sleep better, and drop bad habits such as smoking.

The next section is about his sexuality: how his reproductive system works, sexual problems (from impotence to premature ejaculation), sexually transmitted diseases, birth control, and fertility.

The final section will help you and him if he does get sick, with anything from prostate problems to heart disease.

Share the Facts

Once you're well informed about male health, you can pass along that information at strategic times. When he has a specific complaint, hand him an article or book about possible causes. Don't just tell him the answer. You're not his mother. He'll get more out of it if he digs a bit for the solutions.

Men feel most comfortable discussing athletic injuries ("red badge of courage syndrome"), so start with solid advice on those aches and pains. If he participates in a sport that requires running, for example, buy him a copy of *The Healthy Runner's Handbook* by Lyle Micheli, M.D. If he opens the book looking for help with his aching knees, he'll find that and much more, from recommendations on reducing the likelihood of injury to suggestions for improved nutrition.

Your bookstore and library have many resources. If he likes to cruise the Web, he can find tons of good health information. Look for reputable sites sponsored by medical organizations, universities, or patient advocacy groups. The list of sites at the back of this book is a good place to start.

At the back of this book are "Share Sheets," quick summaries of the most important information about a number of male health issues. You can copy or remove a sheet and hand it straight to your significant other.

Work on Problems Together

Nearly any ailment can be addressed more successfully when you both work toward a solution. Medical problems you have as a couple, from infertility to premature ejaculation, can't be solved without cooperating, but teamwork is just as helpful for other health problems, too. I've even seen men recover more quickly from major surgery because their partners are actively involved in it.

One way to work toward mutual health is to go to the doctor together. If you go with him to his doctor, you don't have to—and probably shouldn't—do the talking for him. Just listen and offer an occasional comment when appropriate. You've probably noticed things about his condition that he hasn't—or at least hasn't thought to mention. Likewise, invite him to go with you when you have a checkup. This allows him to spend time in the medical system without being the focus of attention. He can get used to being in a doctor's office; he can be exposed to matter-of-fact medical care and become more aware of your needs and concerns. You also get the opportunity to model good use of the medical system by drafting a list of questions to ask the doctor, bringing along pertinent information such as old medical records or notes you've made about symptoms, and participating in your care. We'll talk more about these techniques in the chapter on routine health care.

Another thing you can do together is exercise. Studies have shown that

Great Idea, Honey!

Ultimately he won't change unless he owns the process. All along the way you need to convince him that the ideas are his. This may sound cynical or manipulative, but we're interested in results, right? Until an idea belongs to someone, it will never be embraced. Here are some ways you can make him feel in charge.

• Instead of reminding him that he should be going to the doctor, get out your date book and ask him when he'll be seeing the doctor so you can plan your schedule around it.
• Make a ritual of buying him a new toothbrush every month; it's a subtle reminder to use the toothbrush he has.
• Ask him to go shopping for groceries. Provide a list but give him some room to shop. For example, ask him to look for a low-fat version of a particular kind of cheese.
• Ask him to take a child to the doctor. One reason men are so unfamiliar with medical care is that women typically take care of the family's needs.
• Buy him reading material that makes him an expert on the subject. Even better, a computer program offers a particularly male way to approach solving a problem.
• Request that he explain the reasons for a healthful behavior to the children. You know, something like, "Honey, you're an expert on this. Would you tell them why they should eat their broccoli?"
• Brag about his knowledge of health subjects in front of friends. Healthy behavior should be considered expertise, not remedial care.

people are far more likely to stick with an exercise program if they have a partner. If you two hit the sidewalk together, you'll both stand a better chance of walking regularly. In the upcoming chapter on nutrition, I'll suggest that you cook together, too; it's the best way to become aware of what's in the foods you're eating.

You can also work together to compile records about your health. In recent years this has become much more important. The days when a family saw the same general practitioner throughout their lives are over. Today most people switch health care providers frequently, as they change health plans, jobs, neighborhoods. Records can be scattered among several medical specialists' files, too. You should have copies of everything and keep those records throughout your lives. How important is keeping your own records? I have a friend who moved four times while his children were growing up. When it came time for his oldest to go off to college, he was shocked to learn that the family practice where his daughter had been immunized as a baby had disposed of her records after ten years—some seven years previously. Passing her precollege physical became a real trial.

Also get him involved in compiling his family's health history, and the sooner the better. Doctors are constantly adding to the list of diseases known to run in families. As we'll discuss later, diseases as diverse as diabetes and prostate cancer appear to have a significant genetic component. Knowing whether his heritage presents a risk offers the opportunity to anticipate problems and head them off before they become serious. It's not always possible to find out from the written record what ailed Uncle Billy. It's important to interview elders and record what they can recall. This is a great use for a computer, an approach most men find interesting and satisfying.

In most families the female head of the household makes health care arrangements for the rest of the family members. Do what you can to share that responsibility with him. You'll have more luck getting your husband to handle his own health if you first ask him to take part in managing the health of the children. At least, talk with him about their checkups, immunizations, and so forth. Once again he'll be exposed to health care issues without being put personally on the spot. He's also more likely to become aware of how his behavior models behaviors for the children: Like father, like son. I've seen more than a few guys who wouldn't lift a finger for themselves but would climb mountains for their children.

Help Him Bond with Other Men

One of the best ways for men to learn about health issues is by talking with other men. Of course, most men have avoided the subject around other men all their lives, so you'll have to help him find a group of like-minded guys with whom he can feel comfortable.

He doesn't have to get naked or beat drums in the woods. On the simplest level he could attend a seminar on cholesterol at the health club. If he has a particular problem, he could seek out a support group. When he sees that it's okay to talk about health problems with other men, one of the biggest barriers to male health—fear of admitting fallibility—will be behind him.

Another kind of men's group that can present informal opportunities to talk about health is a sports group. You can help him find one. Nearly every community has basketball leagues for adults. Try the local YMCA. Check with a local bicycle shop about group rides, organized for every level of rider from newcomer to seasoned racer. A health club may also be a good place to hang out with the guys. (By the way, when he becomes intensely involved in an outside activity, you may find he's off shooting hoops when you'd rather he be home helping Junior with his algebra. Make sure you arrange for your own time away from family responsibilities. This will not only help him place an appropriate value on his recreation but also make him more responsible when he is home.)

It's also very important for men with health problems to receive support from other men who've stood in their shoes. Most cities, for example, have chapters of the prostate cancer support groups, called Us Too or Man to Man. The group in my area meets in my offices at least once a month. There are similar meetings of men who have lived through potency problems, prostatitis, and, of course, alcoholism. This probably sounds a little odd to you since it's generally women who depend on each other for support through hard times, but men increasingly are learning to lean on one another. Ask his doctor about local organizations. Other sources of leads are local hospitals and the reference desk at the library.

Talk About Health

Finally, try to make health a more frequent topic of conversation. Bring it up at the dinner table, while driving somewhere, or during an evening walk. Chances are you're much more skilled at identifying and describing health problems than he is. As he gets used to talking about his health, he'll grow more comfortable with the topic and he'll gradually become better at identifying and describing health problems.

A major part of my campaign for men's health has been to demystify the male body so it becomes a normal topic of conversation rather than taboo. Most people would be amazed by my family's conversation at the dinner table. Hey, if my sons want to know what happened at work that day, it's likely to include penises and prostates. One way I've tried to bring male health into the open in my public speaking has been to use a set of rubber testes to demonstrate a self-exam. They've been with me to countless conferences and into dozens of radio and television studios. My testes have even been to the White House! I'm fond of saying that I have the most famous testes in America.

My point is not to be crude. To the contrary, I look forward to the day when people can say "penis" or "prostate" in polite conversation as easily as they would say "heart" or "brain." They're all parts of the human body that need to be cared for. If we can't talk about our bodies, it's not likely that they'll get the attention they need. If your man can't talk about his body, how will he communicate with his doctor?

Talk not just about health problems but about health enhancement. Present health not as something given to him at birth that fate may take away but as something he can build. Men love to build things. They like weight lifting because they like to build up their bodies. It's only a small mental step from building muscle (the exterior he presents to the world) to building the entire body.

If he wouldn't relate to body-builder imagery, perhaps he'd like to think of his health as an investment in the future. Together you're building a retirement account by salting away part of what you earn, but a successful retirement depends on much more than money. It's at least as important to build a health retirement account, and it's never too soon to start saving. Health savings bear compound interest just like bank accounts. Healthy behaviors will prevent many problems later on, and you'll also recover more quickly and completely from those you can't avoid. Today's investment in health will help him accumulate the energy and strength to enjoy retirement to its fullest.

* * *

Let's sum up the general approaches you'll be taking to help him change his ways. First, find out where he is along the route to making a change. Learn everything you can about his health issues. Share the facts and help him learn more for himself. Work on problems together. Finally, help him think positive. In the coming chapters you'll learn how these general principles apply to specific behaviors, and you'll learn lots of other techniques and approaches, too.

Help Your Father and Your Son, Too

The "man you love" can be not only a husband or significant other but also your father, father-in-law, or son. It's never too early or too late for all the men in your life to start taking better care of themselves. If they don't, you may someday be saddled with caring for two generations of men with chronic health problems at the same time.

Actually, men of all ages have many health concerns in common. The processes that lead to hardening and clogging of the arteries begin in the teens. Thus the typical teenager's diet, loaded with saturated fat, can be just as damaging to him as it can be to his father. On the other end of the age span, even old men can reverse heart disease with a combination of a very low fat diet, exercise, and relaxation, says Dean Ornish, M.D.

Young and old men are even more likely than middle-age men to benefit from doing testicular self-exams regularly. Testicular cancer is most frequent among men in their late teens to their mid-twenties. The incidence then drops off and rises again after fifty. All men should be doing testicular self-exams regularly, but particularly those under thirty and over fifty. (Later I'll describe how to do this simple self-exam.)

Exercise benefits men at every age. A man in his seventies may not be able to perform at the level of a twenty-year-old, but studies have shown that if he exercises, he'll increase his level of fitness at a similar rate. In fact, old men who take up strength training increase muscle mass almost as quickly as young men do. And the protective effects of that muscle—especially for heading off falls and protecting against osteoporosis—are even greater for older men.

Of course, the approach you're using with your husband or significant other will have to be changed a bit for your father as well as your father-in-law. Many older men are actually easier to convince because they've already brushed up against their mortality. As the years pile on, it gets harder to believe you're bulletproof. The enemy for fathers and fathers-in-law is despair, the belief that it's too late and there's nothing to be done. Most of all they need support and encouragement. You can supply some, but the best kind comes from their peers. With retirement, free time looms large. Unfortunately, instead of getting out with friends and swinging at that elusive white ball, too many older people hang around the house, becoming reclusive. Health goes in a hurry in that environment. Help him get out—by driving him, if he no longer can—and look for places where senior citizens gather. Most areas with large retiree populations have senior centers, which usually include tables for bridge or other card games, shuffleboard, croquet, and other activities tailored to folks who want to stay active but are a little past the tennis court.

With your offspring you have the opportunity to establish healthful behaviors at a very early age, especially if you have the cooperation of their father. As with every aspect of childrearing, however, straight coercion isn't the most effective approach. Kids need rules, but "because I said so" probably won't produce a young man with an enlightened approach to his health. Achieving that goal takes an open and frank approach to health discussions, a willingness to listen, and compassion and love. Above all it takes good role modeling. Men who won't take care of their health typically view it as a personal decision. They view their health as their own business and theirs to neglect if they choose to. Actually, fathers have no such luxury. Aside from the fact that his deteriorating health or death may leave his son fatherless, what sort of picture is he creating of manhood? If he won't do it for himself or for you, what about his own flesh and blood? What sort of man is he? Is he unsure of what to say? Point toward the sidebar "Son, Let's Talk."

Health care for males or females has to start at a young age to be fully effective. Sure, a middle-age or older man can make a big difference in his health, but some damage has already been done. We're never too young to take better care of ourselves.

Son, Let's Talk

Topics every father should discuss with his son:
- Self-exams: testes, penis, and skin
- Aerobic exercise: at least thirty minutes of aerobic exercise three or four times a week
- Diet: a low-fat, high-carb diet will build a pleasing physique
- Sunscreens: at least SPF 15 whenever outside
- Smoking: expose the myth that it's easy to quit; stress that smoking stains the teeth, causes bad breath, and decreases physical performance
- Smokeless tobacco: the risks
- Alcohol and drugs: rehearse how to "just say no"
- Dental care: brush and floss twice a day
- Protective gear: for all sports, including a helmet when riding a bicycle or motorcycle
- Safe driving techniques
- Drinking and driving: tell him he can always call home for a ride with "no questions asked"
- Puberty, sex, and relationships
- Risks of unprotected sex: the only safe sex is no sex

In addition, as men talk to their sons, they need to
- recognize their talents and express pride in their accomplishments, which will help build a positive self-image;
- encourage them to talk about problems when they arise rather than keeping them bottled up;
- respect the son's privacy.

4

Routine Maintenance

Who takes care of the cars in your family? Unless you have a pretty unusual operation, the man of the house changes the oil, rotates the tires, and so forth. Even if he doesn't do the jobs himself, he keeps track of when things should be done and sees to it that they are. Men take a lot of pride in their rolling stock and treat it accordingly. They'd never think of letting their cars run very low on oil or grinding the brake pads down to metal.

While the average man lavishes attention on an assemblage of metal, plastic, glass, and fabric, he totally ignores another system that needs maintenance: his body. He runs his body while it's the equivalent of three quarts low. He needs to think of his body as a mechanical system that needs regular tune-ups so it can continue operating at its best. His body is just like a car that needs oil (or, if he's more the home handyman type, a furnace that needs a new filter every month).

One reason men don't think about routine maintenance for their bodies is that they know next to nothing about what makes them work. While the average man couldn't disassemble his car's engine, he at least knows that his engine is a collection of parts that will fail if they aren't lubricated. He knows that the belts wear out and have to be replaced. He doesn't have a similar basic understanding of his body, so he assumes that as long as he doesn't think about it, everything will be fine. For a long time that may be true, since a young man's body will put up with a lot without complaining. Eventually, though, his body will be not a sports car but a junker.

Why do women have a better basic understanding of their bodies? For one thing, when you period rolls around each month, you have to participate in your body's maintenance. Menstruation forces you to check with your body on a regular basis. No doubt it's one reason you're likely to get a Pap smear regularly, whereas he's unlikely to have his prostate exam regularly. Similarly, you do your breast self-exam, but he skips his testicle self-exam. You're used to thinking about caring for your body, and he's used to ignoring his. In fact, most men don't even want to talk about their bodies, as if the whole subject were embarrassing or unwholesome.

Finding Doctor Right

The days of doctor as authority figure—dispensing diagnoses and treatments from on high—are gone. If managed care hasn't finished off this notion at your house, good sense should. Good health care takes two participants (three if you include yourself): a top-notch physician and an involved, well-informed patient. I call this the health care partnership.

The right doctor can be a very important ally in your campaign to see your man live a long and happy life; he's worth looking hard for.

First, look for a doctor who is as interested in helping his patients *avoid* getting sick as he is in healing them if they do. Prevention is always far cheaper, easier, and more comfortable then a cure. Assuming your guy already has a track record of *not* taking care of himself, he must have a doctor who will help him change his ways.

When I was in medical school about twenty-five years ago, prevention was scarcely part of my training. Doctors who saw the light still managed to emerge from that system, but the focus certainly wasn't on prevention. Instead, we were taught how to put broken bodies back together again. Today, nearly every future doctor receives at least some education in promoting health. The medical system is embracing preventive measures too; for example, the governing body for health maintenance organizations (HMOs) recently published guidelines for routine preventive care. So the odds are improving that you can find an M.D. who will concentrate on helping your man help himself.

Of course, even among the enlightened doctors not every one will be a good match for your guy. Some people just click better than others. That's why you should try several different doctors before settling on one.

The best way to "try out" a doctor is to arrange a brief get-acquainted visit. Many doctors will devote a few minutes of their time—from a cordial handshake to a five-minute sit-down—to getting to know you and explaining their approach to medical care. At the least the doctor should welcome you to visit his offices and offer to talk on the phone after hours. It's also worthwhile to call his office and request some brochures, which will give clues to his approach to care. A brief paid office visit for a chat can be a worthwhile investment.

What do you look for when you get there? The framed diplomas prominently displayed in most clinics don't really mean that much. Anyone licensed to practice medicine graduated from an accredited medical school that offered a good education. Those shingles don't tell you whether the doctor took full advantage of the school's opportunities, nor do they attest to his present adherence to the principles he was taught. Frankly, the other documents on the wall—board certification, hospital privileges, society memberships—aren't that hard to get. Look instead for evidence of the characteristics that ought to be displayed by any physician, from family practitioner to brain surgeon. Here are twelve questions to ask during a get-acquainted visit:

1. *Does the doctor value your time?* In general, you shouldn't have to wait more than thirty minutes past an appointment time. If you spend longer than that in the waiting room, you're owed an explanation and an apology (medical emergencies do come up). Ask the receptionist if the doctor usually runs on time, then check to see if the head count in the waiting room matches the answer.

2. *Is his staff friendly and courteous?* Almost without exception the staff a doctor hires reflects his attitudes about how patients should be treated. A drill sergeant at the reception desk does not bode well. Besides, much of your fellow's care will be in the hands of nurses and physician assistants, so he needs to get along well with them, too.

3. *Do the office hours match your hours?* Many people fail to note whether a doctor is available when they can get there. Does the office close at lunchtime when it's easiest for a working man to come? Are there Saturday morning hours? Also, how do you get in touch with the doctor after office hours? How quickly will he respond when paged?

4. *Who backs up the doctor?* Every doctor needs time away from work, so he arranges to have someone else take his calls during that time. For group practices, the partners usually stand in, but a doctor operating solo will have to make arrangements with another. Find out who backs up the prospective doctor and be sure your spouse is equally comfortable with the backup.

5. *Do the doctor and staff offer extras?* Is the waiting area pleasant? In general, there should be evidence that the team genuinely cares about your

well-being and will go the extra mile for you. Besides a pleasant waiting area with fresh flowers and plenty of reading material, look for a ready supply of brochures describing medical problems and solutions. You might also ask if samples of medications provided by pharmaceutical companies are sometimes offered to patients.

6. *Where are medical tests done, and how do you get the results?* Having tests such as X rays done in the office is convenient, but it's generally more expensive. Also, who analyzes the results? A general practitioner may be capable, but the specialists in a laboratory almost certainly will be. Wherever the tests are done, you should receive results, positive or negative, by mail or by phone.

7. *Are both of you welcome in the examination room?* Any doctor worth his salt realizes that someone with a spouse doesn't have a health problem alone; it affects both of you, and the chances for success are much better if you're both involved.

8. *Does the doctor listen well?* This may be the most important medical skill, especially when the patient is a guy who's reluctant to open up and has a hard time describing his problem. The doctor should let your guy speak uninterrupted during the interview, then ask questions. The doctor should give him his undivided attention (a sure bad sign is talking with one hand on the door knob!). Also, the interview should *always* be done when the patient is fully dressed so the two can meet as equals.

9. *When it's the doctor's turn to talk, does he seem eager to explain?* One of a physician's most important roles is to educate the patient on how to take care of himself. Look out for doctors who use medical jargon to give themselves exclusive control over care. The doctor should choose language that will help both of you understand everything fully. Sometimes a written handout or brochure is better than a verbal explanation. Written materials can provide a lot of important details. They also give you a written record of complex instructions. So expect good up-to-date handouts where appropriate.

10. *Does the doctor provide "high touch" as well as "high-tech" care?* The latest medical technology can be very helpful, but medical care requires empathy and compassion, too. During your get-acquainted interview, notice whether the doctor makes solid eye contact with your guy, a sign of social skill.

11. *Does the doctor take extra continuing medical education (CME) courses?* Some CME work each year is required to maintain a medical license, but a doctor who puts in the extra effort (and expense) to exceed the minimum shows a commitment to staying on top of his profession.

12. *Does the doctor suggest trying the safest, least-expensive options first?* There are numerous ways to treat every medical problem. To get a good feel for a doctor's general approach, ask how he prefers to treat mild hypertension (high blood pressure). If he mentions trying changes in diet and exercise first, it's a good sign. If a drug name comes up instead, look elsewhere.

Health care ought to start with a family practitioner who will work with your partner to improve his health, teach him how to look out for serious problems, work as the front line in detecting diseases, and recommend and monitor treatment by specialists if that becomes necessary. A urologist, of which I am one, deals primarily with male problems, but his specialized skills aren't necessary for day-to-day care. And what about the gender of your guy's doctor? Most men will be more comfortable talking with and being examined by another man, but there are certainly plenty of exceptions to that rule. One of my associates is a female, and she has no problem with seeing men; indeed, she even does worksite screenings. It is a matter of whom he's most comfortable with.

How to Prepare for the First Full Visit

After you've chosen the doctor, if it's been more than a year since your man's last routine examination, schedule one. But before that visit, your guy has some work to do. Even the most skilled and caring physician is only half of the partnership. If your man is to hold up his end of the partnership, he has to make some preparations at home. You can help him arrive for his first full checkup fully equipped to participate. Also, you and he can take care of many details beforehand so there's lots of time during the visit for good interaction. I've also included a Share Sheet (at the end of the book) about preparing for the exam. You might pass along a copy to the new patient so he'll understand what to do beforehand.

Well in advance of the visit, contact all the health providers he's seen in the past and ask for copies of his medical records. Although some of the larger clinics seem to have forgotten this, records are the patient's property, and providers should be willing to hand over copies for a nominal charge. X rays are an exception, but he should at least be able to borrow them. If he's used one pharmacy for some time, it might also be helpful to ask for a record of the medicines that have been prescribed. At the least he should bring any current prescription medications with him to the appointment. When he arrives with a thorough record of the past, time that would have been spent inquiring about that past can be devoted to other topics.

Call the receptionist and ask if any forms can be filled out in advance and whether any test samples, such as blood, could be taken and analyzed beforehand so the doctor can explain the results during the visit. It should be possible to schedule the tests for a weekend.

Be sure he brings along a detailed family history of illnesses. I'll talk more in the next chapter about compiling one. A family health history will help your doctor determine his risk factors.

Help your man make a list of any problems he's had with medications. Any severe reactions will be part of his medical records, but he might not think it worth mentioning subtler problems (for example, an upset stomach from an antibiotic). Write them down anyway. Nothing is too silly to bring up, just as there's no such thing as a stupid question.

Help him make a list of current health complaints and any questions he'd like answered. Most patients—male or female—seem to develop amnesia as soon as they enter an examination room. A list miraculously restores memory.

Find out if he needs to avoid eating the morning of an appointment. Some tests, such as those for diabetes and cholesterol, may require an empty stomach.

What Will Happen During the Exam?

You're probably already familiar with most of the regimens involved in a physical exam, but there are a few differences between the men's and women's versions. Let's run briefly through what is likely to happen so you can be a well-informed coach.

Preliminaries

Before he even sees the doctor, a nurse or physician assistant will check his weight, pulse, and blood pressure. Even though these are simple tests, you can help improve their accuracy by a little advanced planning. Many men have high blood pressure in the doctor's office but not elsewhere because the experience makes them anxious, which can raise both blood pressure and pulse rate. (It's called "white coat syndrome.") He'll be less anxious if he knows what's going to happen during an exam. One simple way to reduce

Joe's List

Here's an example of the kind of list your man should bring with him to a routine checkup.

Health problems of relatives
- Older brother takes cholesterol-lowering drugs.
- Father has had coronary bypass surgery.
- Mother has an underactive thyroid gland.

Personal health complaints
- Insomnia—spouse complains about my snoring.
- Thirsty much of the time, despite drinking lots of coffee.
- Back hurts after sitting for extended periods (office and car trips).
- Occasional hemorrhoid flare-ups.

Medications
- Take one aspirin each day.
- Can't sleep when taking decongestants and become agitated.

Questions
- What is this gray spot on my cheek under my right eye?
- How do I examine my own thyroid gland?
- How can I get rid of hemorrhoids?
- Should I be taking vitamin E?
- Do eggs really raise cholesterol?

anxiety: Is he worried that the doctor's scale will show he's gained weight? If he weighs himself in advance, he'll be a lot less anxious when he climbs on that scale—and when his blood pressure is measured immediately afterward.

When a man has a high blood pressure reading at the doctor's office, it's a good idea for him to stop by the local fire station a few days later and ask a paramedic to check his pressure. When he is under less stress, his pressure may read normal.

A blood pressure reading has two parts. The systolic is the pressure inside the arteries when the heart pumps, and diastolic is the pressure between beats. When discussing blood pressure, we place the systolic number over the diastolic, like division, and say, for example, "One-twenty over eighty."

Any blood pressure reading over "normal" is worth working on. If your guy's in the "high normal" range, his doctor probably won't (and probably shouldn't) recommend drugs to bring it down, but he should make changes in his diet and exercise. Even most cases of mild high blood pressure can be brought into the normal range through lifestyle changes. Readings in the moderate and higher groups should prompt quick action. Drugs might be in order initially, but weight loss and exercise might eventually enable him to get along without the medicine.

Ranking Blood Pressure

What sort of blood pressure results should you be hoping for? For most men the lower the figures, the better. A healthy blood pressure reduces the risk of stroke, heart disease, and damage to a variety of organs. Here's how most doctors rank blood pressure readings.

	DIASTOLIC	SYSTOLIC
Optimal	under 80	under 120
Normal	under 80	120 to 129
or	80–84	under 129
High-normal	85–89	under 139
Mild hypertension	90–99	under 159
or	under 99	140–159
Moderate hypertension	100–109	under 179
or	under 109	160–179
Severe hypertension	110–119	under 209
or	under 120	180–209
Extreme hypertension	120 or over	210 or over

History and Consultation

Before asking your partner to undress, the doctor should sit with him and discuss his background and current health concerns. This is where a prepared health history and a list of questions come in handy. The doctor should ask about personal matters, too—including your spouse's sex life, whether he smokes, whether or how much he drinks, and how things are going in general.

This conversation will be a watershed. A really skilled doctor will be able to get him to talk freely and comfortably, forming a warm and supportive relationship. And you *know* that's no small feat! I leave it to you to decide whether your being in the room makes that more or less likely to happen.

The Once-over
After the history and consultation, the doctor will ask your guy to change into an examination gown; he'll probably step out for a minute while this goes on. Upon returning he'll start at the head, working downward to:
• check the eyes (for acuity, voids, or dark or black spots in the field of vision, damage from high blood pressure, and, if he's older, glaucoma);
• look and whisper into the ears (for infection and hearing problems, nothing personal);
• inspect the tongue and gums for signs of oral cancer (his dentist should be doing this, too);
• listen to the neck (for bruits that may be obstructing blood flow, a sign of impending stroke);
• check the thyroid gland (for swelling or lumps);
• examine his skin—especially the face, ears, shoulders, and the backs of his hands (for signs of skin cancer);
• listen to his chest (for heart sounds and lung congestion, crackles, or wheezes);
• massage his chest (for lumps that might suggest breast cancer);
• probe his abdomen (for liver size, kidney and spleen problems, and abnormal masses);
• massage areas in the neck, arm pits, and groin (for swollen lymph nodes);
• check his abdomen and groin (for hernia);
• examine his testicles and penis (for cancer or other abnormalities including warts and sores);
• tap arms, knees, ankles, and toes (for reflexes);
• check muscle strength;
• prick his arms and legs (for sensation) and move them (for signs of weakness).
He didn't forget the rectal exam; he'll get to that in a few minutes.

While this process is going on, your man should feel free to ask why the doctor is doing certain things. A basic skill of doctors is to be able to explain what they're doing while performing routine exams. Besides, people who enjoy their work are usually pleased to talk about it.

Tetanus Shot

Shots are no one's favorite part of a physical, but there's a good chance your guy is overdue for a tetanus booster. It is needed only once every ten years, but for that very reason it's easy to lose track. When I ask patients when their last tetanus booster was, I usually get this response: "Gosh, it seems like a few years ago, but I can't remember." Although tetanus (lockjaw) is rare these days, the reason is inoculation. One of the merits of finding (and seeing) the same primary care physician is that your records will be there to say for certain what you need and when. Otherwise, you need to keep track yourself.

Diagnostic Tests

Once the basic physical exam is over, there will be a variety of tests, depending on your guy's age.

Digital Rectal Exam

Beginning at forty he should have a digital rectal exam (DRE). The doctor will ask him to lie on his side or bend over a table; then he will insert a gloved, lubricated finger into the anus to check the prostate for lumps, hard spots, and overall consistency (a process called palpation). DRE is *the* front-line test for early detection of prostate cancer. At the same time the doctor will examine the rectum for abnormalities (hemorrhoids, for example) and will remove a small amount of stool to be tested for blood (a hemocult test, which may indicate colorectal cancer).

Quite a few men dread a DRE more than any other part of the physical. They'd rather have surgery. But for most the procedure is far more humiliating than it is uncomfortable. (A DRE should never hurt; if it does, he should say, "Stop!") A good doctor will try to help him relax, which makes the test much easier. Taking a deep breath and exhaling slowly may help, as will focusing his attention on something else. In some cases I even recommend that a man take a warm bath before coming in for an exam. When I was on the Gary Collins show, he asked me why DREs aren't done first, to get them out of the way. If it sounds better that way, ask for it. It's a simple enough thing for a doctor to arrange.

Colon-cancer Screening

Once a man (or woman!) hits fifty, he should have a more thorough exam of his nether regions with a sigmoidoscope every five years. If he flips out at the thought of having a finger inserted in there, the thought of a medical instrument is likely to bring on real anxiety. Take my word for it, though, it's not so bad. The instrument is small and flexible—by now all the old rigid sigmoidoscopes should have been melted down as scrap—and the exam doesn't take too long. He should feel good about taking care of this important test; the risk of dying of colorectal cancer is 80 percent lower for men who have sigmoidoscopy even once.

While a person of average risk should have this test every five years, the American Cancer Society recommends that if a sigmoidoscopy turns up polyps (noncancerous growths), the person should have a colonoscopy (full colon examination) at the time of diagnosis and within three years of polyp removal. If that test shows no further polyps, the person is then considered of average risk and goes back to the five-year interval. People with a family history of polyps or colorectal cancer are considered to have a high risk, and the ACS recommends they have exams as early as puberty.

Tuberculosis Test

Ten years ago the medical community thought tuberculosis was beaten, but it came back. Treating it has become more difficult, too, as new strains of the disease are resistant to antibiotics. Men over forty should have a Mantoux skin test every five years. TB is once again on the decline, mainly because of increased awareness.

Electrocardiogram

Starting at forty he should have an electrocardiogram (EKG) to measure the rhythms of his heart and to reveal signs of any previous heart attack. (Many people are surprised to learn that they can have a heart attack without knowing it.) The EKG reveals how well his ticker is working by measuring the electrical pulses emitted each time the muscle tissues of the heart contract. After small areas of skin are shaved, electrodes are taped to his chest, arms, and legs. Signals picked up by these electrodes can be printed out or recorded for replay.

EKGs are often done during exercise since his heart may work fine until it has to work hard. During a "stress test," he'll walk on a treadmill at a gradually increasing rate and slant. As his body demands more oxygen, the EKG will be able detect whether the heart is getting enough oxygen.

A stress test is particularly important before a man takes up exercise after years of doing one-arm potato-chip lifts on the couch in the front of the TV. Nearly everyone—even people recovering from heart attacks—can benefit from exercise, but it's important to know how much exercise and what kind. A stress test will help his doctor find out. Otherwise, EKGs aren't necessary until he reaches his forties and then only every four years. However, he should have one EKG in his thirties to establish a healthy baseline to which later tests can be compared. By charting the changes in his heart's action, his doctor can see trouble coming long before it becomes life-threatening. If he develops a health problem that may be related to his heart, it could be vital to compare an old EKG to a new one. Keep a copy of the baseline EKG—most newer equipment can produce two original printouts—and bring it to each health evaluation. A man who has heart trouble ought to carry copies of his EKGs with him when he travels, just in case.

Chest X Ray

Chest X rays aren't a standard part of a physical, but they can be very helpful in diagnosing heart enlargement and lung problems such as emphysema and chronic bronchitis. Most of the time chest X rays are given to check for lung cancer. If he smokes, I strongly suggest that he regularly have a chest X ray. Although lung cancer is one of the most frustrating cancers to treat, medical science is making progress. In the past few years pioneering techniques have been developed for removing small lung cancers. *Small* cancers. If a tumor grows to any significant size, there's not much we can do, so early detection is vital.

Urine Test

A urine test tells quite a bit about his waste-processing system. To get a little technical, it reveals kidney function (protein, acidity, and concentration), infection (nitrates), diabetes (sugar), liver function (bilirubin), cancer and stones (blood), and whether the body's store of sugar has been used up (ketones). All these readings help eliminate the possibility of serious, though uncommon, diseases. A man's urine usually reveals as well that he isn't drinking enough water (he should be drinking eight to ten glasses a day). Most of the time the results of a urine test should be available by the end of the office visit.

Blood Tests

A blood test is the single best source of clues to what's going on in a man's body. From a single sample we can look for evidence of prostate cancer, check cholesterol (the stuff that plugs arteries), measure sugar levels (to see if he's on the verge of full-blown diabetes), and, as needed, diagnose several other health problems. Let's look briefly at the three most common blood tests.

Beginning at fifty (forty if there are risk factors such as a family history of prostate cancer) and up to age seventy, all men should have their prostate specific antigen (PSA) levels checked every year. After age seventy it depends on life expectancy, so a man should discuss it with his doctor. Prostate cancer killed about 42,000 men in 1997. The PSA test is the best way to detect prostate cancer early, when treatment is most effective. A PSA test detects between 85 and 90 percent of all prostate cancers. (Fortunately, DRE tends to catch the cancers PSA misses; that's why doctors recommend the combination.)

The PSA test measures a substance made only by the prostate. A PSA measurement of 4.0 or more almost always means something's wrong with the prostate—but not necessarily cancer. Prostate enlargement, infection, or irritation, or even recent ejaculation can boost PSA into the 4.0-to-10 range. (Sorry, but amorous activity is strictly off limits for forty-eight hours before the test; you can help by reminding him of this important detail.) If his results are in this range, the first step is to repeat the test since PSA levels can vary as much as 45 percent between tests. If the level is still elevated, the trick is to determine whether he should have more expensive and involved tests, such as ultrasound-guided needle biopsy. For more information about possible further tests, see chapter 20, "Prostate Problems." PSA testing can also be used in more sophisticated ways to refine prostate cancer risk. We'll talk more about PSA velocity and free PSA in chapter 20.

Another important blood test is a full cholesterol test, more accurately called a lipid profile. In addition to total cholesterol it reveals levels of low-density lipoprotein (LDL) cholesterol, high-density lipoprotein (HDL) cholesterol, and triglycerides. LDL is often called "bad" (or "lousy") cholesterol because it forms plaque on artery walls. HDL, "good" cholesterol, appears to combat the accumulation of plaque. Triglycerides account for about 95 percent of the fats stored in the body. Though triglycerides alone don't appear to be very dangerous, recent research has shown that when both triglycerides and cholesterol are elevated, risk of heart disease goes up significantly.

Your guy's maximum acceptable cholesterol levels are determined by his level of risk for heart disease. Just being male is one risk factor. Others include a family history of heart disease before fifty-five, cigarette smoking, high blood pressure, HDL lower than 35, diabetes, history of stroke or arterial disease, and obesity. If all he has going against him is his male sex, his total cholesterol should be less than 240 and his LDL less than 160. For men with two or more risk factors, though, total cholesterol should be less than 200 and LDL less than 130. In any case, HDL should be between 35 and 65. With HDL, more is better. This test is more accurate if done in the morning after fasting since the previous evening.

A serum glucose measurement (done when he hasn't eaten since the previous day) reveals diabetes and other problems with carbohydrate metabolism. In a healthy person the hormones insulin and glucagon strictly regulate the blood's level of glucose, the body's primary energy source. Glucose levels below 60 or above 115 should be further evaluated with a glucose tolerance test.

It takes several days to get the results of a blood test. Unless your partner arranged to have the sample taken before his physical, he'll learn the results by phone. If there's a problem, of course, he'll return for another visit. However the results are delivered, ask for a copy and add it to the health record you are keeping. Occasionally, repeat or additional tests may be recommended. Your guy should be given a thorough explanation as to why the test is called for and what sort of preparations he needs to make.

The Second Opinion

When is a second opinion in order? *Anytime* a doctor recommends surgery or another risky or very expensive procedure and *anytime* either of you isn't satisfied with the diagnosis or treatment. You're not second-guessing the doctor, you're doubling your guy's chances of getting the right treatment. Any conscientious doctor will be relieved to have his conclusions confirmed or questioned because in the long run a second opinion is in the best interest of both patient and doctor.

If the doctor resists a second opinion or seems offended when another doctor disagrees with him, it's time to find a new health partner. Urge your man to stand up for his rights; do it yourself if you have to. It's not just the principle—it's his health.

As your guy becomes more and more informed about his health, he'll eventually be able to offer a second opinion himself. Help him learn to take advantage of all opportunities to learn about his health. Encourage him never to hesitate to question. In the end, no matter how many doctors he consults, he should make the final decisions about treatment.

5

Flashing Red Lights

Male folklore contains many stories about women who misinterpreted or shrugged off warning lights on the dashboard of the car. The woman is credited with saying things like "Gee, honey, it wasn't blinking" or "I planned to tell you about it when you got back from your trip." The ending of most such stories is terrible harm done to the car, to the complete surprise of the woman.

Such tales are born in the locker room and don't ring true. Women are far more likely than men to pay attention to warning signs and then do what must be done. In my practice I see plenty of evidence that *men* are the ones who overlook the obvious. When I examine a man who has a testicle the size of a grapefruit, I know the tumor didn't get that large overnight. Sadly, a self-exam could have detected it even when it was very small. Self-exams could save so many lives.

Self-exams help people pick up signs of trouble so they can have a much better shot at early detection when treatment is often easier, cheaper, and more effective. Even at best, your man sees his doctor for a routine exam only once a year, but he sees himself every day!

Before I tell you how the basic self-exams are done, let's talk about your guy's family health history. Since many health problems have a genetic link, a family health history will help identify the self-exams about which he should be especially diligent. If he knows he's at risk, he'll be more motivated.

Digging Out His Family History

At first most men don't want to know their family health history. They're afraid they'll learn they have a "bad gene" that's doomed them to develop a disease. If your guy thinks of his genetic inheritance as a potential curse, start by clearing up his misconceptions. The vast majority of genetic mutations don't make a disease inevitable; they just increase the likelihood. Usually the increased risk can be offset by changing your habits and having regular screenings.

Genes are linked to more than four thousand diseases, most minor or only slightly more likely to occur because of the gene. On average each of us has the DNA for ten of these genes. Unfortunately, it's not yet practical to test broadly for such genes (a possible exception is testing the siblings and children of people with certain forms of breast and colorectal cancer). For the time being, family health history offers the best insights into risks. Your guy should investigate the health histories of his brothers and sisters, parents, aunts and uncles, and grandparents, but it's not always easy to learn about the health of others. If you think your man's generation is reluctant to talk about their plumbing problems, you should talk to the one before. There's not much chance that Granddad openly discussed his colorectal or prostate cancer.

Once someone has died, it gets even harder to find out their health history. Even if you look at a death certificate, the official cause of death may be just a complication of an underlying health problem. For example, if a person bedridden with cancer develops pneumonia and dies, the official cause of death can be listed as pneumonia. Of course, a person who has cancer can die instead of a heart attack. Someone can survive a heart attack, then die years later in an unrelated car accident. And so on.

Because official records don't tell the whole story, it's important for your spouse to talk to his living family members and record who has had what. If your man's father is still living, that is the most important interview. There's a lot that every son doesn't know about his father (and vice versa). But men will talk, given the opportunity; I see it happen all the time.

Usually it doesn't work to just sit down in the living room for a talk. The men will probably accomplish more if they talk while doing something they both enjoy, like fishing, golfing, or hiking. If you have a son, suggest he come along, too; his presence may help bring down the barriers. Encourage your guy to fit the occasional health question into the banter that accompanies such activities. He may be surprised by what he finds out—and it could save his life.

The women of the family are another source of health information. If your guy doesn't feel comfortable talking to his mom or sisters about their health, it may work better if you do those interviews. If he's willing to give it a shot, encourage him, because it'll be easier for him to get information out of the women than the men. It'll be a good warm-up for the talk with Dad!

As he talks to his relatives, what health problems should he ask about?

Prostate Cancer

A man whose father had prostate cancer has a two-and-a-half times greater risk of developing it. If his father or uncle developed cancer before age fifty-five, his chance is one in two. That's a significant risk, but it's still far from a death sentence. As long as the cancer is discovered before it moves out of the prostate, the chance of successful treatment is very, very high. Men with a family health history of prostate cancer should begin having both digital rectal exams and PSA blood tests at age forty. They should also be including in their diets foods that may reduce the risk or prostate cancer (notably soy products; see chapter 20 for information about the prostate).

Testicular Cancer

Cancer of the testes also has a strong genetic link. Since the disorder is most common among males eighteen to twenty-five, and again after sixty, many middle-age women should worry about their sons and fathers even more than their spouses.

Men whose fathers have had cancer of the testes are four times more likely to develop it themselves than is the average man. The genetic tie is even stronger between brothers; when one gets the disease, the other's risk is nearly ten times greater than the average male's. With each succeeding generation, genetically based testicular cancers appear more likely to start at an earlier age, to affect both testes, and to spread to other organs. Another indicator of risk is having testicles that failed to descend before age two. You know if your son did, but what about your husband and father-in-law?

Early detection is even more important for testicular cancer than prostate cancer because it often grows rapidly. Found early, testicular cancer can be cured completely and relatively easily. If there's a history of the cancer in your guy's family, it's really important that he do regular self-exams (see below).

Colorectal Cancer

Many cancers of the lower digestive tract have a genetic link. A family history of colorectal cancer increases his risk, but he can lower that risk with a diet low in saturated fats and high in fiber, and with regular screenings starting at an early age. While most men should have a test for colon cancer starting at

Health History Checklist

When talking to blood relatives about their health history, ask about the following disorders. Note how old the person was at the time of diagnosis. Also write down if the person has been overweight or has smoked.

Heart disease
High blood pressure
High cholesterol level
Angina (chest pain)
Stroke
Colorectal cancer
Lung cancer
Prostate cancer
Testicular cancer
Breast cancer
Skin cancer
Other cancer
Emphysema
Diabetes
Allergies
Depression
Schizophrenia
Alcoholism or drug addiction

age fifty, the American Cancer Society recommends that people with a family history of polyps or colorectal cancer be screened as early as puberty.

For certain forms of colorectal cancer, tests are being developed that identify the genes that do the dirty work, but these expensive tests aren't yet widely available and definitely aren't called for unless there's a high risk of that particular type.

Other Diseases with Family Ties

Of the other diseases with known or suspected familial links, many are preventable, curable (with early detection), or both. It pays to know the genetic road map and take a few simple steps to avoid potholes.

Many forms of diabetes run in families, but a low-fat diet and regular exercise can help head off diabetes and control it without insulin. Knowing he's at risk and acting accordingly can help him avoid ever getting the disease.

Although no one should smoke, men with parents who've had emphysema ought to be the first to quit.

Heart disease and high blood pressure run in families, too. High cholesterol is also an inherited problem, one that's particularly dangerous in men; half of men with familial hypercholesterolemia die by age sixty.

You probably don't know that vulnerability to some forms of skin cancer can be passed from generation to generation. If a parent or grandparent has had skin cancer, it's especially important to be diligent about sunscreen, wear a hat and long sleeves outdoors, and do self-exams.

Self-Exams

To explain the purpose of self-exams to your guy, you might compare them to the radar detectors of the cold war's early-warning system; they make it possible for him to detect any incoming attacks so he can stop them before they even reach him.

If the word "exam" brings back bad memories from school days, he might like to call these "self-checks" instead. Your guy may also find a "partner-exam" more appealing than a "self-exam." A partner-exam is a logical part of a caring relationship, and he'll see right away that it can lead to interesting possibilities!

Testes

Although we've made great advances in treating testicular cancer—over 90 percent of cases can be cured—early detection makes the job much easier, and chemotherapy and lymph surgery are avoided. Unfortunately, few young men are aware that testicular cancer is the number one solid tumor in males under forty. Even athletes, who are relatively aware of their bodies, can fail to notice a growing tumor. For example, by the time Scott Hamilton's testicular cancer was diagnosed in March 1997, the tumor was the size of a grapefruit and had spread to his abdomen. After chemotheraphy and surgery, however, the figure skater will probably recover fully.

A testicular self-exam is unquestionably the most vital self-exam for men under forty. Every father should teach it to his son along with the facts of life. After sixty, incidence of the cancer rises again, and so does the importance of the self-exams.

Simply put, even if your guy is a good patient, he doesn't see the doctor often enough to have a decent chance of catching testicular cancer before it's too late. It's his responsibility to find it.

Every male who's reached puberty should examine his testes at least once a month. The best time is when he's in the shower because the warm water relaxes the scrotum. Of course, there's no reason why you can't help. To check testes, grasp each one between your thumb and first two fingers, with your thumb behind. Gently run your fingers around the circumference of each testicle looking for lumps or hard places. The testicle should feel like a small hard-boiled egg without its shell. In back, where your thumb is, you may find a lump called the epididymis, but the rest of the surface should be smooth and pliable. A lump or hard place is plenty of reason for him to see a doctor *immediately*. This is not something to report at his next physical.

By doing the test every month—the first of the month, say, since it's easy to remember—he'll get a sense of what's normal, so any change will immediately be obvious. Again, any change is a call to action; he can't get to the doctor too soon.

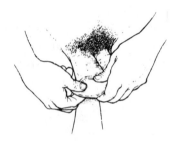

The Penis

While he's still in the shower, a man should take a minute to examine the skin on his penis. It should be smooth and have no red areas. As they age, many men develop brown spots or small flesh-colored bumps. Neither is a cause for concern unless there's a rapid change.

He should note any sores or lumps and, as long as there's no rapid change, mention them to his doctor at his next checkup. Anything that develops quickly merits a phone call to the doctor. A sore could be something as simple and unthreatening as an irritated hair follicle. Or it could be a sign of a sexually transmitted disease. Or it could be the beginning of penile cancer. You two can be the investigators, but let his doctor be the judge.

Skin

Once a month he should also check his skin for signs of skin cancer. The average man has about a 40 percent chance of getting skin cancer (somewhat higher than a woman's risk simply because he spends more time outdoors in the sun). There are three main types of skin cancer. Basal cell and squamous cell carcinoma can usually be cured without too much difficulty, but malignant melanoma can be deadly.

Over the past forty years all types of skin cancer have become much more common, perhaps because of the thinning of the Earth's protective ozone layer. Many skin cancers begin when skin—specifically a gene called p53—is damaged by the ultraviolet radiation of the sun.

As is the case with most health problems men inflict on themselves, sunburns are usually more accidental than intentional. He just doesn't think about how long he's been in the sun or about simple preventive measures like sunscreen of at least SPF (sun protection factor) 15, a hat, and long sleeves. You can help by setting a good example.

However, neither you nor he can change history. Chances are he spent a lot of time in the sun when he was a boy and young man. Since significant damage may already have occurred, self-exams are important. A 1996 study estimated that self-exams could save nearly two-thirds of the 7,200 lives lost each year to melanoma.

You both should be checking your skin at least once a month. Because some areas are difficult to see, partner-exams are even better than self-exams. Some skin cancers develop in areas that have been exposed to the sun, but, surprisingly, melanomas are more likely to be on the trunk and legs. So check each other from the soles of your feet all the way to your scalp. It's time to see a doctor if either of you has a sore that doesn't heal or a molelike growth that has one or more of these characteristics:

- Asymmetrical (not round) shape
- Borders that are irregular
- Color variation across its surfaces
- Diameter bigger than a pencil eraser

Just remember A, B, C, D.

Breast Cancer

Most people think that only women get breast cancer. Not only do men get it, but it's exactly the same disease, except that men are more likely to get it near their nipples since they have less breast tissue elsewhere.

Although breast cancer occurs much less often in men than in women (about 1 man in 100,000), it does happen. I diagnose a couple of cases each year, and for me it has struck much closer to home. A few years ago, after reading my first book, my father detected a lump in his breast. Fortunately, he noticed his cancer early when it was curable. As a woman you're well aware that early detection is very important with breast cancer. Because most men aren't aware that they should be doing breast self-exams, they're unlikely to catch a tumor early. The result is that for men the cancer is more often lethal.

Once a month your guy should be doing the same self-exam that you do, but with extra emphasis on the area around the nipples. For starters, retraction of a nipple, dimpling, or discharge are early warning signs. He should also feel each breast for lumps with the pads of his fingers, using the left hand to examine the right breast and the right for the left. The tissue should have the same consistency throughout, there should be no changes from one month to the next, and gentle pressure should not cause pain.

Oral Cancer

Many people mistakenly believe that it's safer to chew tobacco than to smoke it. The rate of oral cancer is four to six times higher among men who use smokeless tobacco. In a man whose vices are limited to smokeless tobacco, it takes decades for mouth lesions to become cancerous, but when alcohol is added, cancer develops much more quickly.

You can point out to your guy that baseball players, many of whom use oral tobacco products, have unusually high rates of mouth, throat, esophagus, and stomach cancers. The minor leagues have already banned chewing tobacco, and the majors are gradually moving in that direction. The Los Angeles Dodgers, for example, now prohibit players from carrying tobacco products when in uniform.

Although cancers of the mouth and throat are very rare among people who don't use tobacco products or alcohol, no one should ignore a persistent sore in the mouth. Checking is a simple matter of running the tongue around the gums to search for persistent sore spots. Any spot that doesn't begin to heal in a few days should be examined by a doctor or dentist. (By the way, your dentist should be examining both of you for potential cancers every time you have a checkup.) Oral cancer is a miserable way to die.

Thyroid

Cancer of the thyroid, a butterfly-shaped gland just below the Adam's apple in the neck, is far more common than most people imagine. About fourteen thousand new cases are diagnosed each year—nearly three times as many in women as in men. Fortunately, when it's detected early, thyroid cancer is usually curable. You can easily check each other for thyroid problems using a simple glass of water, or he can check himself with the water and a handheld mirror. Watching the area just above his collarbone, ask him to tilt his head back and take a swallow. Watch for any bulges or protrusions (besides the Adam's apple). If you notice any, he should go to the doctor immediately.

Lymph Nodes

Lymph nodes, the focal points of the lymphatic vessels that return fluid from tissue to the blood, are sensitive indicators of infections and cancer. You both should regularly check the lymph nodes in your neck, armpits, and groin for swelling and tenderness. The lymph nodes will be tricky to find when everything is fine, but a swollen node will stand out and demand attention. If either of you finds one, see your doctor to find out what's causing the inflammation.

Pulse

A normal pulse is between 45 and 70 beats per minute, with a lower number in men who are in good physical condition. An abnormally low or high pulse can mean that there's a problem. Your man should be checking his pulse every month or so when he first wakes up in the morning. He should report a change of more than 20 points to his doctor. He should also be on the lookout for irregularities in his pulse, which may be normal but could signal one of a group of conditions called arrhythmia. A pulse check will also be an important part of his exercise program, because he'll be checking to see whether he's in the zone for safe, effective conditioning. By the way, as he becomes fitter, his morning pulse rate will drop.

Practice taking your own pulse before showing him how. Place your index and second fingers on your neck between the side and front. Feel for the indentation where there is a strong pulsing. Count the beats for ten seconds, then multiply by six to calculate your pulse rate per minute.

Blood Pressure

Nearly a third of men over eighteen have high blood pressure, and it's never too early to bring it under control. We should all check our blood pressure every few months. Many pharmacies offer free measurement, or you can stop by the local fire station. If your guy's blood pressure is above normal at his checkup, though, it's especially important that he measure it regularly. Buy him a blood pressure cuff (called a sphygmomanometer). It will cost less than $30. (The gift may not seem very romantic until you consider that it expresses your interest in seeing him live awhile.) By measuring his blood pressure at different times of the day, he'll learn how much of the time it's elevated. He may even get an idea of what is causing it to go up; for example, is it elevated only at the office? See chapter 4 for a chart about interpreting the results of a blood pressure test.

Teach Him How to Measure His Blood Pressure

1. Wait for at least thirty minutes after exposure to stimulants that raise blood pressure: caffeine, eating, exercise, and cold. If he's taken a decongestant, his blood pressure may be elevated for hours.

2. Suggest that he use the bathroom if necessary.

3. Ask him to sit in a chair next to a table positioned so he can rest his arm comfortably on the tabletop with the palm up. He should then relax for five minutes.

4. Wrap the cuff around his upper arm so that its lower edge is about an inch above his elbow and the tubes are positioned to the inside and directed toward his hand. Tighten it enough that it won't slide off.

5. Place the gauge on the table so he can see it easily.

6. Slip the cup ("microphone" end) of the stethoscope up under the cuff on the inside and put the earpieces in his ears.

7. Tighten the valve on the squeeze bulb. Pump the cuff up until the gauge reads about 180.

8. Loosen the valve slightly so that the pressure begins to bleed off by 2 or 3 millimeters a second.

9. When the pressure drops between 150 and 120, he'll begin hearing a tapping noise. The pressure when he first hears that sound is his systolic pressure.

10. As the pressure slowly bleeds off, the tap will gradually become a swishing noise and then a less distinct tap. The pressure at which he last hears any noise is his diastolic pressure.

Potency

If he's having a problem with erections, won't it just be obvious to both of you? True, but a simple self-test can help find the underlying cause. Problems with erections are always a symptom of another physical or emotional problem.

While they sleep, all potent men have two to four erections lasting fifteen

---

to thirty minutes. We're not even aware of them unless we happen to wake up when erect to urinate.

To find out if he's having nighttime erections, snugly wrap a strip of postage stamps (no need to spring for first class here; any denomination will do) around his penis and glue one end to the other. If he has an erection during the night, the swelling will break the stamps along a perforation. Lack of nighttime erections often portends a serious physiological problem such as heart disease or diabetes. I'll talk more about how erections tie into other health problems in chapter 15.

Learning to Listen to His Body

While self-tests uncover quiet problems before they become noisy, many ailments announce their presence loud and clear. You probably find it difficult to believe that anyone would ignore these blaring sirens, but never underestimate a man's power of denial. Here are some of the serious symptoms for which he should be on the lookout.

The Seven Warning Signs of Cancer

According to the American Cancer Society, everyone should watch for seven warning signs of cancer. Here they are, with a few examples.

1. A change in bowel or bladder habits such as a thinner stool, a change in color of urine or stool, or a change in frequency

2. A sore that doesn't heal

3. Unusual bleeding or discharge in his ejaculate, in his stool, or in his urine, or coughing up blood.

4. A lump or thickening anywhere on his body such as under an arm or on his breasts

5. Indigestion or difficulty swallowing

6. Obvious change in a wart or mole

7. Nagging cough or hoarseness

Chest Pain

Chest pain, especially during exertion, is a sign that the arteries can't supply enough blood to his heart. This pain, called angina, can range from a sense of tightness in the center of the chest to very severe pain that may radiate to the neck or down the left arm. Angina is a sign of heart disease—an early warning sign of an heart attack down the road.

A number of less dangerous conditions, including heartburn, can mimic angina. Only an electrocardiogram and blood tests can tell the difference for sure.

Many people are able to reduce their angina by losing weight, stopping smoking, getting regular exercise (as directed by a doctor), and changing their diet. If these steps don't work, drugs or surgery can help prevent a heart attack. There's much that can be done if the man doesn't just shrug off those pains he feels when he runs up the stairs.

Many men do just that, unfortunately. I got a call about a year ago from a woman asking which medication I'd given her husband. I pulled his file and was reminded that the man had seen me for Peyronie's disease (a curved penis), for which I'd prescribed a drug. When I called the woman to answer her question, I learned that her husband had died. I offered my condolences and asked her to tell me more. It turned out that, besides the Peyronie's disease, he had suffered from what he thought was severe indigestion. He had pressure in his chest, even radiating down his left arm, when he ate and at work, so he took great quantities of Tums. He had failed to mention this problem to his primary care doctor when he saw him for the penis problem or to me when he was referred. One morning, the woman woke up, rolled over, and found that her husband was dead of a massive heart attack at age forty-five.

Dizziness, Fainting, Heavy Sweating, and Shortness of Breath

Although pressure or pain in the chest lasting more than a few minutes is one of the most common symptoms of a heart attack, some people have severe heart attacks without feeling as if there's a truck driving over their chest. Other symptoms of a heart attack are feeling dizzy, faint, sweaty, or nauseous. Among older people a very common sign is severe shortness of breath. Far too many people delay seeking treatment because they don't have the classic symptom of chest pain. These other symptoms may, of course, signal other problems, such as asthma or lung disease, but they're always cause for a prompt medical attention. He should call 911 or get to an emergency room immediately because much of the damage of a heart attack happens in the first two hours.

Erectile Dysfunction

A recurring problem with getting or maintaining erections is always a symptom of other health problems. More than half the time erectile dysfunction stems from a physical problem, such as clogged arteries, high blood pressure, or diabetes. Also, more than a quarter of the men who see me for erection difficulties have high cholesterol. Researchers at the St. Louis V.A. Hospital found that about a quarter of all men who see a doctor for a potency problem have a heart attack or stroke within five years. Even when emotional problems are at the bottom of things, a limp penis is still a sign of another problem that should and can be treated on its own.

Stroke

Most men imagine that they would know it if they were having a heart attack, but I find very few can list the symptoms of stroke. Stroke is the leading cause of disability in the United States. Early treatment can greatly lessen or reverse a stroke's effects. The warning signs are:
• Sudden weakness or numbness of one side of the face, an arm, or a leg
• Sudden dimness or loss of vision, particularly in one eye
• Loss of speech or the ability to understand speech
• Sudden severe headache without other cause
• Dizziness, unsteadiness, or falls, especially along with any of the previous symptoms

Diabetes

The most common form of diabetes develops gradually during the adult years. Symptoms become progressively worse until diabetes is full-blown and potentially life-threatening. With a few simple lifestyle changes, diabetes can be controlled or even reversed, but improvement is much easier in its early stages. Your man should talk to your doctor about diabetes if he has two or more of the following symptoms:
• Regular or constant thirst
• Frequent need to urinate
• Fatigue
• Unexplained weight loss

Depression

We all have occasional periods of the blues, but depression is different. Depression is so common and so underdiagnosed in men that I've devoted much of an upcoming chapter to it. Depressed people—and especially men— are unlikely to see their condition as a treatable medical problem, so he's dependent on you—as you are on him—to recognize the signs. He should see his doctor if for two weeks he shows at least one of the first two signs in the following list, and five signs altogether:

- Depressed mood
- Loss of interest or pleasure in usual activities
- Feelings of worthlessness or excessive or inappropriate guilt
- Inability to concentrate or make decisions
- Fatigue or loss of energy
- Appetite change or weight loss
- Sleeping too little or too much
- Jerky or slow physical reactions
- Unusual and persistent pains, such as headache
- Recurrent thoughts of death or suicide

Vision Problems

Although few people have heard of it, macular degeneration is the most common cause of blindness over fifty. About 1.7 million people are legally blind because of it, and more than 11 million show signs. Macular degeneration is yet another example of a health problem that can be stopped if detected early, but it has no cure once it's done its dirty work. If you and your spouse are seeing a skilled optometrist each year for a checkup—as you both should after age forty—he or she should be monitoring for this condition as well as for glaucoma, diabetic retinopathy, and cataracts. Symptoms such as blurred vision, eye pain, rainbow halos, spots, or more severe vision impairment are always cause for a checkup with an eye specialist.

Keeping Track of His Health

If your guy finds a problem through a self-test or through a "flashing red light," he should record it. Memories are not nearly as accurate or permanent as a written record. Just as important after recording a health event is paying attention to it. He will come up with more details about the experience. And as he writes down the information, the whole experience will seem more real to him. The act of recording a health event reinforces the whole string of good health behaviors we're hoping to encourage.

His notes should have answers to questions like these: What did the pain or symptom feel like? When he had the symptom, what else was going on? Did something he ate bring it on or make it worse or better? Did he have other symptoms (even ones that don't seem related)? What treatments did he try (this includes both prescriptions and over-the-counter medications and even simple changes in his behavior, such as lying down)?

Questions to Help Him Open Up

If I ask a male patient about a pain, he's likely to reply, "It just hurts" or "It hurts all over." Men spend most of their lives trying to ignore or cover up health problems rather than becoming skilled at identifying and describing them. You can help your man develop a health vocabulary by asking a few strategic questions:

"How long have you felt this way?" He'll probably reply that he doesn't know, but you can help him along by supplying a time line. For example, "Was it there when we went to the movies on Saturday night?"

"Have you had these symptoms before?" He may not recall a previous episode until you pique his memory.

"Is it constant, or does it come and go?" This helps him concentrate on what he actually feels.

"Is it getting better, worse, or staying the same, and what causes the change?" Considering the progress of the problem helps him get in touch with it.

"Has it disturbed your sleep?" This gives him a specific situation to concentrate on.

"Does it worry you, or is it just irritating?" Men seldom consider the emotional impact of physical problems. This gives him the opportunity to express his feelings about his problem.

"Is it similar to a toothache or more like slamming a finger in a door?" Comparison may be easier for him than describing whether the discomfort is dull or sharp. And the extreme example—the finger in the door—may help to lighten the situation up a bit. Not much hurts more than that.

Getting him to write about his health is a formidable challenge. Journal keeping doesn't seem to be a male thing. The trick is to make the task as convenient as possible. If he's a dedicated computer user, he may like to record health information on the same program he uses to plan future appointments and deadlines. Similarly, the daily planner most businessmen carry can readily be used to keep track of past events. However he keeps the record, he should bring it along when he goes to the doctor.

I'm forever telling men that there's no excuse for being surprised by a heart attack or other problem. If your man pays attention to his family medical history, listens to his body, and has regular checkups, he and his doctor should be able to monitor his condition and head off the kind of surprise no one wants.

Part II

"All the Things You Are"

6

Beyond Killer Biceps

He loves sports, but he won't exercise. Riding the couch for a Saturday afternoon of football won't inspire him to toss a ball with the kids, let alone walk or jog. As a matter of fact, it's more likely to spur a stroll to the cupboard for potato chips and then a late-afternoon nap.

Why doesn't he see the irony? Because he learned at an early age that exercise is for the few. Football was played by thirty of the biggest, most talented guys in his high school class; he watched. At the college level it's even worse; only 3 percent of men participate in an organized sport at the average university. In school he was taught that exercise is for the elite.

Among the few who did make the football team, how many still play the game in their forties? Many once-muscled torsos now sink into belt lines. One reason is that school athletic programs are designed to win games, not to develop either a healthy attitude toward exercise or skills for lifelong sports.

Because men believe that athletic activity is the domain of *young* men born with *a special capacity* to be strong, fast, and fit, they don't believe exercise will make much difference for them. Sure, ask a man if he thinks that exercise is healthful, and he will give it lip service. Who's to argue when scientists from the Cooper Institute report in the *Journal of the American Medical Association* that men who exercise die at half the rate of those who don't? When it's been proven that exercise can reduce blood pressure and the risk of diabetes? But such facts still inspire only about half the men ordered to exercise for recovery from a heart attack to do it.

Not only does he think exercise isn't for him, but he's convinced that it's unpleasant. Men associate exercise with aching muscles ("no pain, no gain"), pushing the limits, and extreme effort. Here the problem is that most men who do start exercise programs set unreasonable goals. This leads not only to injury but also to giving up. Reasonable goals allow interim successes that keep motivation strong. (By the way, since the word "exercise" has poor connotations for him, you might do better calling it "conditioning" or "training.")

To start and continue an exercise program, he needs two things: the right kind of motivation and reasonable thresholds. Fortunately, these are two areas where you can make a real difference. If you do, you will win twice: the first time because your own exercise habits will improve, and the second because the man you love will be healthier for it.

After his triumphant return season to the NBA, Michael Jordan said, "What made the difference was my family's support, my wife and my kids. My wife pushed me every day. When I didn't feel like getting up and working with my trainer, she set the alarm and made sure I got up."

The Right Kind of Motivation

If he believes implicitly that only the talented and young exercise, and he won't take it up because it's good for him, what *can* motivate him?

For men, the best motivation is good company. Studies of exercise program compliance have shown conclusively that the single best predictor of success is having a regular workout companion. Early in an exercise program it's particularly helpful to work out with his most understanding companion: you.

When people exercise together, they can carry each other over the humps of difficult days. One day you may feel like it when he doesn't, but if you suit up, he won't want to be left behind. Another day the roles may be reversed.

Working out with someone else will also help take his mind off what he is doing. In the beginning, exercise won't be entirely pleasurable, and twenty or thirty minutes can seem like a long time when he's by himself. When there's someone to talk to—and the ability to maintain a conversation without gasping is a measure of the correct intensity—the time flies by.

As he starts to get into shape, you can also help him look for a group of like-minded guys who get together to work out. An adult hockey or softball league, a regular game of basketball at the Y, a racquetball ladder at a health club, a tennis league, a running or biking club—there's bound to be something he likes. There are also coed groups you can join together. One group of ten men has been meeting every Wednesday evening for years. They run ten to sixteen miles, then eat pizza at a member's house and watch a video. What began as a training group for a marathon has evolved into an important part of their lives.

A woman described to me how camaraderie made all the difference for her husband:

> When Jim developed mildly elevated blood pressure in his thirties, our doctor told him to try exercise before resorting to medication. He loved hiking and even bought a bicycle, but he didn't stick with either. They were too inconvenient, and with a house and kids, there was always something else that needed doing.
>
> It wasn't until he got a new job where several of his coworkers bicycled at lunchtime that exercise became a regular part of his life. At first he rode just with them, but before long he wanted to go a little farther and a little faster. Jim found a bunch of guys his age who ride from a local bicycle shop in the evenings. Now he does a hundred miles most weeks, has lost fifteen pounds, and has his blood pressure under control. He's been doing better at work, including a raise and a higher tolerance for office annoyances. He looks terrific, and feeling better and stronger has definitely enhanced his interest in *me*, too.

The second motivation that really works is to include strength training—in other words, weight lifting—in the workouts. A man who takes up exercise tends to go straight to the weight room (whereas women are apt to start out by walking). The prospect of bulging biceps or prominent pectorals appeals to, well, his vanity. He wants to be attractive to you (though actually women are just as likely to be attracted to a winning smile). Even more important, he wants other men to view him as powerful. All jokes aside about ninety-eight-pound weaklings having sand kicked on them at the beach, most men feel the emotional tug of big muscles. We still live in a society where men are rewarded for power, and we still haven't evolved enough from our hunter heritage to make *intellectual* power the whole story.

Luckily, strength training will improve not only his looks but also his health. It's particularly important after fifty-five when it can prevent a debilitating injury by keeping his muscles and bones strong. A story I hear too often goes like this: He hadn't exercised for years. In his sixties, he got up during the night to go to the bathroom, and because his muscles were weak, he fell and was unable to brace himself for the impact. Because lack of exercise had also weakened his bones over the years, he broke a hip. In the hospital, the nursing staff was too busy to get him up and moving often enough. Pneumonia developed, as it will in the bedridden, and that was it. (Even at the end, strength training could have helped since studies have shown that even a few weekly sessions with light dumbbells can help the elderly get out of bed and move about.)

You won't have to sell the long-term health benefits of strength training, though, since he'll want that powerful physique. However, despite the value and appeal of strength training, he should start with a few weeks of an aerobic activity such as walking before gradually adding weight training. For one thing, every weight room session should be preceded by a warm-up session of aerobics in order to reduce the chance of injury. Also, without guidance the average guy will pump iron until he's sore if not strained. Aching or injured muscles are not conducive to sticking with an exercise program. His motto should be "No pain, great gain." Once he's established a moderate aerobic program, arrange for him to work with a personal trainer to get a well-rounded routine. Most health clubs have a trainer on staff. You can also find an independent trainer by calling the American Council on Exercise (800-529-8227); they will provide the names of up to three certified trainers in your area. Look for a trainer who has been certified by the American Council on Exercise, the American Academy of Health and Fitness Professionals, the American College of Sports Medicine, or a similar organization.

Besides companionship and a desire for rippling muscles, what else can motivate him to rise from his easy chair? Though he may be a hard sell on long-term health benefits, some short-term health gains may be more convincing. Exercise will help him:

• **have more sex.** When a group of older men in a study at the University of California, San Diego, took up moderate aerobic exercise four times per week, their rate of intercourse increased 30 percent.

• **be happier.** Aerobic exercise is now recognized as an effective treatment for mild depression and as an adjunct to the treatment of more serious depression. It also appears to reduce anxiety and help people cope with stress.

• **stay young.** A Washington University study found that men in their sixties who exercise have the cardiovascular health of men in their twenties who don't.

• **sleep better.** Exercise helps men, particularly older ones, fall asleep in half the time and awaken less often during the night.

• **be smarter.** When people who exercise were tested for reasoning, memory, and reaction time, they performed better (by about 20 percent) than sedentary folks.

- **get sick less often.** Men who exercise take fewer sick days from work. If he's ambitious, he'll like this.
- **be more regular.** Exercise decreases the time it takes the body to fully process food, so men who exercise are less likely to become constipated.
- **ease his back pain.** The American Academy of Orthopedic Surgeons recommends physical activity and specific strengthening exercises to relieve chronic back pain.
- **avoid cumulative trauma syndrome (CTS).** People whose jobs require repetitive motions have one-quarter the risk of being diagnosed with this disorder if they exercise vigorously.
- **be a better role model.** If he won't exercise for his own good, maybe he will to show his son or daughter a healthful lifestyle.

Even though these benefits are attractive and relatively immediate, if you present them as a demand, he'll just dig in his heels. And as we've discussed, nagging is unlikely to be effective and is guaranteed to be unpleasant for you. Probably the best approach is to offer exercise as a solution when he complains about one of the above problems—along with a measure of sympathy, of course.

Starting Right

As millions of failed exercisers can attest, taking up exercise is much easier than sticking with it, particularly the way men are inclined to approach it. I already mentioned that, given their druthers, men will head first for the weight room, and return home with sore muscles and one more bad experience with exercise. Unfortunately, their second choice—running—is almost as bad.

Unless he ran when he was younger and has gained little weight since then, running invites failure. First, for an unfit person, there's no such thing as running at a moderate pace. Just moving from a fast walk to a run will elevate his heart rate beyond the level appropriate for aerobic fitness. He may have the grit to suffer through the gasping and become fit enough to run well. More likely, though, he'll conclude that he "hates running" and head back to the TV.

Moreover, when a guy takes up running in his middle years, carrying an extra ten or twenty pounds around his middle, he's asking for injury. His knees and ankles aren't as supple and forgiving as they once were, and he's putting more stress on them. Even if he weren't middle-aged and a bit overweight, his odds of injury would be high. Among the 26 million American runners, at least 80 percent eventually experience an overuse injury.

Not that running is bad exercise. It's hard to beat for effectiveness, convenience, economy, and pure pleasure. I run and love it (although I have to admit that my back has recently limited my mileage). Running is just not a good choice for someone who's beginning an exercise program. Far better that he start by walking, an activity that's equally convenient and economical but far less risky. Walking at a vigorous pace—at least four miles per hour—offers much of the benefit of more punishing sports, and the rate of injury is very low.

I suspect you don't need to be sold on the value of walking since it's women's number one fitness choice. As convinced as you might be of its benefits, though, think twice before trying a direct sales pitch. Walking is just not macho. Instead, just do it: Go for a walk and invite him along. Ask him to take the dog for a walk. Buy him a fancy lawn mower that he *walks behind* rather than rides on. (The lawn tractor may have done as much to compromise the fitness of American men in the last half of the twentieth century as any other technological development.) Hey, why not take a vacation and take a walk on the beach?

How much aerobic work does he need? I recommend three or four sessions of at least thirty minutes per week. After thirty minutes, the body preferentially consumes fat to provide energy, so more is better.

For some people, especially those in agreeable climates, walking can fill their aerobic needs. Most of us, though, do better with a variety of aerobic activities. A treadmill or exercise bicycle will drive many people to tears of boredom if it's their only form of exercise. But as a rainy day alternative, machines work well—especially if there's a TV to watch or a way to read while doing it. I read journals on the treadmill or exercise bicycle, and it really helps me keep up with medicine.

Indeed, variety is in itself an important way to ensure that he'll stick with exercise. Some activities inherently offer a fair amount of variety. Outdoor walking, running, and bicycling, for example, have scenery going for them. If your local climate has frigid winters or brutal summers, check out the early-morning walk hours at your local mall, offering a view of enticing store windows. Some people like the low-stimulus, meditative quality of swimming and exercise machines; others simply find them tedious. So help him fit his choices to his tastes. Doing something he doesn't like will lead to failure.

Set Realistic Goals and Monitor Progress

What he would like to accomplish with exercise may be quite different from what you see as a sensible goal. Recall that lowering blood pressure, heading off diabetes, and reducing heart disease risk are not likely to appear on his short list of expected benefits. Even feeling better and more energetic are a bit abstract for the average guy. He has something more concrete in mind, such as losing a certain number of pounds, adding inches to his biceps, or developing washboard abdominal muscles. Fortunately, looking better and being healthier can go hand in hand, especially when he's aiming for a realistic goal.

First and foremost, discourage him from using the bathroom scale to measure progress and success. In the early months of an exercise program it would tell a misleading story. A balanced program of aerobic exercise and strength training reduces body fat and increases the size of the muscle tissue. Since muscle weighs more than fat, his weight may increase at the beginning, even though he's making great progress. Eventually he will lose some pounds, but they shouldn't be the focus of his concern in the beginning.

Concentrating on weight also enforces another misleading male behavior: the weigh-in. As a regular at a gym, I can't recall ever seeing a guy weigh himself *before* a workout. The sacred pilgrimage to the scales comes at the end, after he's sweat heavily and showered, if not after a spell in the steam room, hot tub, or sauna. During extended, vigorous exercise an average guy can shed two to three pounds of water in the form of sweat, especially when intentional sweating is added at the end. (Football players have been known to lose ten pounds during a game.) The scale tells a story of dramatic success, but he can't stay dehydrated indefinitely. Those pounds will return in a few hours as he drinks to replace the lost water.

Better ways to measure progress are a belt and a mirror. Each notch of the belt accurately records increased health because abdominal fat has been shown to be a significant predictor of a variety of health problems, including heart disease and diabetes. He'll like this measure of success because he wants to banish that potbelly. The notches are a concrete measurement and will follow one another relatively quickly as his body fat declines and posture improves. Clothes are a similar way to measure progress. Nothing is more rewarding than trying on new pants in a smaller size or slipping into a pair you haven't been able to squeeze into for years. One way to celebrate his progress is to bring his favorite old clothes out of the back of the closet.

As he cinches in that belt, you can help him develop a better overall sense of his body by encouraging him to use the mirror. When looking in a mirror, most males don't look below the razor line, afraid of what they'll see. As his body mass begins to shift away from his middle, let him know that you're liking what you see. He'll begin to sneak peeks and will like what *he* sees. He may even develop the ability to honestly assess his own condition, which forms a cornerstone of taking care of himself.

In the meantime, though, record keeping helps. Work with him to develop an exercise plan and then write down what is actually accomplished. The plan should include at least thirty minutes of aerobic exercise (more is better) at least three days a week, stretching, and two or three strength-training sessions (at this point note muscle groups rather than specific muscles—for example, legs, arms, shoulders, abdomen, back). He'll find it motivating to look back and see how far he's come.

If a day is missed, just get back on track. Constant skips mean the threshold is too high or motivation is still lacking.

Finally, a note of medical caution: Any man forty or older who's been mostly sedentary for an extended time should have a physical exam before taking up exercise. A man with a heart condition, for example, needs to approach exercise with caution and under a doctor's supervision. Your guy could have one of those without knowing it—until he tries that ten-mile run. Likewise, if he gets hurt exercising, encourage him to see a doctor. Knee problems are particularly common among middle-aged men taking up exercise, and they won't go away without proper foot and leg alignment (through shoe insoles) and strengthening exercises. Injuries happen, but they shouldn't be taken as a sign to stop. They just suggest that it's time to get help and get back in action.

While I have stressed setting realistic goals, I purposefully haven't set down any magic numbers. The right goals will emerge as he develops a better sense of his physical self. Exercise in and of itself can help him do that. When he uses his body, he will become more aware of it. With a little subtle guidance and love, he can come to consider it an ally. He'll learn his own strengths and weaknesses, and how to make the best of them. Not only will he feel better about himself, but he'll also take better care of himself. You'll both be happier for that.

Getting Beyond the Excuses for Not Exercising

HE: It's not the right time to start.
YOU: You'll always be busy, so this is as good a time as any. If you wait for the perfect time, you'll never get started. I'll help you find the time.

HE: I'm too tired after a hard day's work.
YOU: You could get up earlier or work out at lunch. Let's tour that new health club near your office.

HE: Do you expect me to look like Arnold Schwarzenegger?
YOU: Uh, uh. Muscle tone, not size, is what's important to me and you.

HE: It hurts too much to exercise hard enough to do any good.
YOU: At the right intensity, you should be able to hold a conversation. That's not hard.

HE: Exercise is boring.
YOU: Let's get some cool bikes and join the crowd in the park. It will be fun.

7

A Steak and Potatoes Man

I agree with the old saying "Food is love." Familiar, lovingly prepared foods are some of life's greatest comforts. Unfortunately, many men's comfort foods are very high in fat and sugar. Not only do rich, fatty, sweet foods taste great to them, but they bring back childhood memories. My mother used to cook thirty lamb chops at a time: ten for Dad, ten for me, eight for my younger brother, and two for herself. Our mothers served eggs for breakfast every day, urged us to drink quarts of whole-fat milk, and made pot roasts and apple pie for dinner. They thought these foods were good for us. Such a diet was never healthful, but at least men used to burn up the heavy meals working in fields or factories. We know much more about nutrition today, but too often we eat the same way. How can you help him grow beyond his culinary childhood?

Fundamentals of Male Nutrition

Putting aside for a moment the question of how, let's talk about what. What *should* he be eating? For the most part the same foods that make you healthy make him healthy: minimal dietary fat; moderate amounts of protein; lots of complex carbohydrates such as bread, cereal, rice, and pasta; a lot of fruits and vegetables. However, male nutrition is different from female nutrition in some important ways. Certain bad dietary habits will harm him more, and he needs more of certain nutrients and less of others than you do.

Protein

If you suggest reducing the amount of red meat in a man's diet, he'll probably say he works hard and plays hard and needs protein to build strong muscles.

True enough, but odds are he eats half again as much as he needs. It's hard to live in America, get the calories you need, and be deficient in protein. A plate of pasta, not even counting the sauce, has a quarter of the 63 grams recommended daily for men twenty-five and older. One chicken breast takes him more than halfway there.

Protein quantity is basically not an issue, but quality does matter. He should be choosing the protein sources lowest in fat: the leanest red meats, skinless chicken, egg whites, and lots of seafood. There is one other protein source worth mentioning, although he may consider it a dirty word: tofu. Not only is it a great source of protein, but it also contains genistein, which may help protect men from prostate cancer.

You may have chuckled when I mentioned the word "tofu," knowing that there's no way your spouse would eat the stuff. I have a friend who still maintains he doesn't touch tofu, despite the fact that I've sat across the table from him while he eats it in Chinese food. Hard as it may be to believe, the description "bean curd" on the menu didn't offend him, and the waiter pronounced it "dough-foo." So my buddy is an unknowing tofu consumer.

Dietary Fat

Nearly ten years into the fat revolution, everyone knows dietary fat is bad. Particularly bad is saturated fat, found primarily in red meat and dairy products and also in coconut and palm products and cocoa butter. Dietary fat raises blood cholesterol levels, which in turn increase the risk of heart disease, the leading killer of men.

Fat also increases the risk of prostate cancer, which is now the most common cancer in America (250,000 new cases each year) and the second leading cause of death in men after heart disease. This link was first suggested by studies of Chinese and American men. In America the death rate from prostate cancer increased from 15 per 100,000 in 1930 to 25 per 100,000 in 1990. During the same time in China, the rate stayed steady at less than 1 percent of the American rate. An obvious difference between the countries is that the American diet is much higher in fat. And, indeed, Chinese men who immigrated to America and adopted the American diet lost their advantage.

Further studies have found that Chinese and American men have almost the same chance of having a very small prostate tumor. (Autopsies of men who died from other causes have revealed that about 30 percent of men over fifty have small prostate cancers that were undetectable by noninvasive means.) Something causes the insignificant cancers in American men to become big problems. Recent research points directly at dietary fat. Human prostate cancer cells grafted into mice develop much more rapidly when the mice are fed a high-fat diet. Fat may or may not cause prostate cancer, but it dramatically influences whether that cancer will become life-threatening.

Chinese and Chinese-American men also face very different risks of getting colorectal cancer, and, once again, fat seems to be the cause. A recent study comparing Chinese nationals and immigrants to the United States attributed 60 percent of the colorectal cancer in men—particularly sedentary men—to their increased consumption of saturated fat.

In the next chapter we'll discuss other reasons that your man should avoid fat and how you can help him actually do it, but even with the support of health facts, you'll find this a tough battle. Changes have to be made little by little, almost meal by meal.

Fiber

Among the virtues of a high-fiber diet are reduced risk of various colon problems (constipation, hemorrhoids, diverticulitis, and cancer), lower cholesterol, 40 percent lower risk of heart attack, avoidance or control of diabetes, and, of course, the fact that it's not fattening.

A man should eat at least 30 grams of fiber a day, but the typical man eats less than half as much. Good sources of fiber include beans (9 grams per half-cup), bran and bran-based breakfast cereals (as much as 15 grams per half-cup), whole grain breads (3 grams per slice), potatoes (4 grams each), peas (4 per half-cup), and fruit (4 for an apple or pear, 3 for a banana or orange, 3 or 4 for a cup of berries). Many products on the supermarket shelves make claims about fiber. In numerical terms a "good source of fiber" or "contains fiber" means 2.5 to 4 grams per serving; "high in fiber" or "rich in fiber" means at least 5 grams per serving.

Fiber is relatively easy to introduce into a man's diet, but he shouldn't add too much too quickly. It takes the digestive tract time to adapt to the new regimen, and hurrying may have a side effect that's unpleasant for both of you: gas. Increasing fiber content over several months will do much to preserve domestic harmony.

Water is particularly important when adding fiber to his diet. He should drink at least eight cups per day, both to aid in the digestion of the fiber and to keep his urinary tract working in good order.

Minerals

Men need more zinc than women do. Zinc increases immunity for both sexes (for example, speeding recovery from colds), but men also need it to produce healthy sperm and, some studies have suggested, to maintain sex drive and a healthy prostate. Good sources of zinc include wheat germ, oysters, chicken, and lean red meat.

On the other hand, men need less iron than women do. Excessive iron may be a factor in heart disease for men since high levels of an iron-related substance are found in the blood of men who have had heart attacks. As long as he doesn't have a fondness for liver or a heavy raisin habit, it's probably not necessary for him to intentionally limit iron intake, but he should avoid supplements that include iron as well as breakfast cereals fortified with iron.

You've probably already increased the calcium in your diet to protect you from osteoporosis (brittle, thinning bones), but you may not know that he should, too. About 20 percent of osteoporosis cases occur in men. Calcium also lowers blood pressure, reduces LDL (bad) cholesterol, and prevents kidney stones. (People who already have kidney stones should consult with their doctor about calcium.) Good sources of calcium include low-fat or nonfat dairy products, fortified orange juice or breakfast cereal, and greens such as collards and kale.

Magnesium helps keep the heart muscles working correctly. Good sources include seafood (especially shrimp, clams, and crab), sunflower seeds, spinach, peas, beans, and almonds.

Potassium plays a role in controlling blood pressure and can be found in potatoes, raisins, bananas, and orange juice.

Should he restrict the salt in his diet? Some people with high blood pressure (particularly those on medication) can cut their blood pressure significantly by reducing salt intake. For others it makes no difference. If he doesn't have high blood pressure, he doesn't have to take extreme measures, but it's probably best to avoid adding salt to food. Most of us get far more (about 4,000 milligrams per day) than we need (2,400 milligrams per day), much of it hidden in processed foods.

Antioxidants

Antioxidants are chemicals in foods that neutralize free radicals—highly reactive oxygen molecules—helping to prevent heart disease, several cancers, complications from diabetes, cataracts, and even some aspects of aging. Vitamins C and E and beta-carotene are the best-known antioxidants, but several others—such as selenium and other members of the carotenoid family—are also worth accenting in his diet.

Too little vitamin C clearly harms health, but large doses don't seem to prevent disease as much as Linus Pauling and others have claimed over the years. Recent studies have found that vitamin C does have an important role, though—it makes vitamin E work much better. Aside from citrus fruits, good sources include broccoli, cantaloupe, cauliflower, and strawberries.

If vitamin C's performance has been spotty, vitamin E's track record has improved with age. Since 1990, repeated studies on large groups of men and women have shown that vitamin E intake well in excess of the recommended amount (which is 15 international units for men) lowers the risk of heart disease by about 40 percent, on average, and of prostate, breast, lung, and colon cancer by around 20 percent. Recently, it has even been found to delay the symptoms of Alzheimer's disease. What's more, no negative effects have been found from increasing vitamin E intake to 400 international units. Unlike every other nutrient discussed here, it's practically impossible to get enough vitamin E through food. Vitamin E is most concentrated in fatty foods such as oils and nuts. To get even 100 units, he would have to toss down seven cups of peanuts, which would pack a whopping 4,000 calories. So a daily supplement of 400 international units makes sense.

Beta-carotene, like vitamin E, blocks the oxidation of LDL (bad) cholesterol, helping to prevent damage to coronary arteries, and has been associated with reduced risks of several cancers. As a supplement, though, beta-carotene's performance has been less stellar than vitamin E's. Two recent studies sponsored by the National Cancer Institute found no benefit from beta-carotene supplements and even a small negative finding for people who smoke. It may be that supplements don't work as well as eating foods rich in this beta-carotene: yellow and orange fruits and vegetables such as peaches, apricots, carrots, and squash, and green, leafy vegetables such as spinach, broccoli, and mustard greens.

Other close relatives of beta-carotene—a group known as the carotenoids—have been associated with reduced risk of a number of ailments. Tomatoes, for example, contain lycopene, and men who eat a lot of tomato-based foods (only cooked tomatoes) are much less likely to develop prostate cancer than those who don't (up to 45 percent less for those who eat ten servings per week). For men who do not like tomatoes or are intolerant of the acidity, supplements are available. Likewise, spinach contains lutein, another potent carotenoid antioxidant.

Finally, there's selenium, an important antioxidant much in the news lately. The selenium content of food depends on the soil in which it is grown, so there are wide variations regionally. Patterns of a number of cancers and heart disease seem to correspond to these regional variations. One preliminary study found that selenium supplements reduced risk of cancer, including prostate cancer. The problem with selenium is that we need it in very, very small amounts, and too much can be toxic. At this point I can't recommend supplements, and it's difficult to know which foods to eat to increase selenium in the diet. But selenium is worth keeping an eye on as researchers look at it more closely.

Other Vitamins

When the rate of prostate cancer is plotted on a map of the United States, it increases slightly from south to north. The difference may be vitamin D. The body makes vitamin D when it's exposed to sunlight. In the South, sunlight is stronger, and it's warmer so there's a greater chance that people are outside. There's still more to be learned about the link between vitamin D and prostate cancer, but men should include some vitamin-D-fortified, nonfat dairy products in their diet. This is particularly true for older men whose bodies don't make vitamin D as efficiently. Incidentally, lest he use vitamin D as an excuse for sunburn, thirty minutes of direct sunshine a day is plenty to synthesize the vitamin.

The last of our essential nutrients may turn out to be as important as any. Folate is a B vitamin found in vegetables including spinach, okra, dried beans and peas, and in fortified cereals. The higher the concentration of folate in the blood, the lower the levels of an amino acid called homocysteine, which is achieving notoriety as a major risk factor for heart disease and stroke. Studies show that men who report eating lots of foods rich in folate have a 20 percent lower risk of stroke than those who don't. Of course, those foods are packed with other powerful nutrients, but folate may well turn out to be one of the most important parts of the package.

In the End, It's Pretty Simple

All the complicated nutrient names—grams of this and international units of that—can sound fairly daunting, but the basic plan is quite simple, and probably quite familiar to you: He should be eating minimal dietary fat, moderate amounts of protein, lots of complex carbohydrates, and lots of fruits and vegetables.

It's best to get the essential vitamins and minerals from foods because foods high in them tend also to be high in other important nutrients and fiber. To be safe, however, he should take a daily vitamin and mineral supplement.

A Man's Place Is in the Kitchen

How do you get him to substitute fruits and vegetables for a big hunk of beef with a potato and sour cream? Obviously not by making a simple swap. You'll just hear the question, "Where's the rest of dinner?" And turning yourself into a "food cop" probably won't do either of you much good—let alone make you happy. I've had the distinct displeasure of visiting households where the female has taken on the role of nutritional policewoman. It never looked as if anyone was having any fun, and I never noticed it working.

As is usually the case with men and health matters, you'll probably have to take the lead. Once again, though, it's really not a bad deal. Not only will you have a healthier, happier partner who spends more quality time with you, but you'll also enjoy the fruits (and vegetables) of your labors with him.

Even before you read the section above, you probably knew a lot more about nutrition than your man does. The reason is that you're doing most of the grocery shopping and cooking. You read the labels and see what goes into the dishes. The average male's mastery of food preparation extends as far as barbecuing burgers and microwaving frozen dinners, so his approach to cooking hasn't had a chance to develop. To raise a man's food consciousness, get him to cook—and not just steaks on the grill. Only when he takes an active role in his diet will he become conscious of what he's eating. Without that awareness, nothing you do will make much difference. Until he faces the fact that he is what he eats, he'll negate your best efforts by laying on the fat at lunchtime, sneaking snacks, and turning business travel into a dietary indulgence.

In the best of all possible worlds he'd be ready to step into the kitchen and share the work (and fun) right now. In the real world, though, it takes some enticement and no small amount of patience to get him cooking. Why not start in familiar territory: the barbecue. Grilled fish and chicken (with the skin removed) are healthful alternatives to the ritual beef. At first you can help him out by preparing low-fat marinades; before long he'll want to develop his own special seasonings. Next, he can learn to grill vegetables and even fruits. Bell peppers, onions, tomatoes, pineapple, eggplant, brussels sprouts, and mushrooms can be grilled on skewers in a cool corner, especially if you steam the firm ones a little for him first. Corn can be wrapped in aluminum foil. Even asparagus does well if cooked gently. Coach him a little if need be, but let him own the process. Then be sure he knows you liked it; there's nothing more conducive to an encore than sincere applause.

As he gets more inventive in the backyard, he'll spend more time preparing in the kitchen. This could present a strain or two. Many avid cooks find refuge and peace in the kitchen, so sharing it with someone else—especially someone who, at least initially, may seem pretty inept—could be a challenge. If this has been your turf, where you call the shots, you may have to bite your tongue when he makes unnecessary messes, and you may get in each other's way. Some couples thrive on working together in the kitchen; others definitely do not. It may turn out that you'll have to spend a little time reading while he takes over in the kitchen.

Another good way to encourage his participation in food preparation is to get him involved in kitchen tasks that involve appliances. Devices such as bread machines appeal to the male love of gadgets, and you'll probably soon find that he's making all the family's bread. Noisy juicers can also be a hit. Knowing what goes into food—even if it's as simple as flour, water, and yeast—will help him better understand what's good for him and what's not.

Let's Go Out Tonight

Eating out, and particularly eating while traveling, can be a real challenge to a healthful diet. Too often those so-called diet plates include full-fat cottage cheese and consider twelve ounces of ground round to be low calorie. There are ways, however, to eat lean on the road. Try making these observations:

• Foods that are mixtures of different things almost always involve a rich sauce. Instead, stick with a piece of fish (broiled), a vegetable, and a plain baked potato.

• If he orders an entrée that has a sauce, he should ask for it in a bowl on the side. He will use a lot less that way.

• Ethnic restaurants can be good or bad. The beans and rice that are Mexican staples are excellent foods as long as they're not cooked in lard and covered with cheese. Likewise, Chinese foods can be great (tofu and broccoli, for example) or disastrous (Kung Pao, for example).

• Pasta is a great choice as long as it's not covered with a cream sauce. Basic marinaras are very lean, and even a meatball might not bring too much fat to the meal.

• Good restaurants often offer tempting breads before the main course arrives. Encourage him to eat plenty—without butter.

• A restaurant is no place to practice for the clean-plate club. If the serving sizes are large, take some home for tomorrow's lunch.

Not until he can see a doughnut as a combination of flour, shortening, and full-fat milk deep-fried in saturated fat and covered with fat-based frosting will he really embrace low-fat living. Only then will he be willing to substitute a bagel or a low-fat bran muffin.

Does he like to brandish knives around? Get him into stir-fries, with lots of vegetables that need to be cut up in tiny pieces. Does he fish or hunt? Buy him a fish or game cookbook. Some men love making complicated dishes for company (dirtying every pot in the kitchen, of course, but at least they're cooking). Would he like to "own" a certain night of the week—say Friday or Sunday evening? You know him better than anyone. What will turn him on to cooking?

"Food Is Love" Revisited

Besides nurturing his culinary expertise, put your own to work and revisit his mom's old recipes. There are many easy ways to lighten recipes so they have a better nutritional profile without much difference in taste. Many low-fat cookbooks are full of ideas. Gradually substitute more healthful ingredients for salty, oversweetened, fat-saturated ones. Learn about lower-fat cooking methods, too. After a while his taste buds will change, and he'll lose his taste for salt, sugar, and fat. For example, if he drinks full-fat milk, switch to 2 percent. A month later buy 1 percent. Later, switch to skim. Once he is used to skim milk, even 2 percent milk will taste disgustingly rich, like cream. Coaxing a man out of his dietary comfort zone isn't easy. It must be done step by step, one serving at a time.

Take advantage of your power as the family grocery shopper. If there are low-fat pretzels in the cabinet instead of potato chips, he'll eat pretzels. Again, make change gradually and moderately, or he'll undo the good when he's on his own. But don't fall into the trap of buying potato chips because you know he likes them and you want him to be happy. Sure, it'll work for the moment, but you have to keep your eyes on the future prize. You want him around for the long run, and there's no time like the present to begin making changes that will help that happen.

In the next chapter we'll talk more about eating strategies such as variety, snacking, timing of meals, and more. In the meantime, though, why not start putting your new nutritional strategies to work? Better yet, put *him* to work— cooking a piece of salmon.

Ten Tips for Improving Male Nutrition

1. **Steam rather than boil vegetables.** Boiling leaches many of the nutrients from vegetables, so they end up going down the drain with the water.

2. **Put salad dressing on the side.** Not only does a small bowl of dressing reduce the amount he uses, it also helps the salad ingredients stay fresh.

3. **Add nonfat powdered milk to skim milk.** It makes it richer and increases the calcium content without adding fat.

4. **Bread and bake chicken instead of frying it.** Baked chicken has far less fat.

5. **Swap mustard for mayonnaise.** The first is nonfat, whereas the second is mostly fat.

6. **Substitute veggies and pretzels for chips as snacks.** Low-fat ranch salad dressing makes a good dip.

7. **Get in the olive oil habit.** Evidence suggests that this mono-saturated fat is king of the vegetable oils.

8. **Avoid fats that are solid at room temperature.** Partially hydrogenated fats, such as margarine, may be just as bad as butter.

9. **Buy him a little refrigerator for his office.** Send him to work every Monday with a stock of low-fat yogurts, fresh fruit, and mineral waters so he won't hit the soda and candy machines so often.

10. **Go wild with herbs.** Dried or fresh herbs, mustards, vinegars, fruit preserves, and cooking wine are better ways to enhance the flavors of foods than salt or butter.

8

There Is More of Him Than There Used to Be

W ay back in a dark corner of my closet hangs the wardrobe of a different guy: the fat me. It's been a long time since I was that guy, but I could become him again anytime. All I'd have to do is slack off and live the way I used to. Oh, I'm no Superman with extraordinary power to resist temptation. I do slip from time to time, but so far I have gotten right back on track.

I've been able to lose weight and keep it off. The average man gains a pound a year between his twentieth and sixtieth birthdays. What makes me different? The love of a fine woman. Even with my medical knowledge about weight management, without my wife's example, encouragement, and day-to-day support, I never would have succeeded. She showed me the way. You can do the same for your man.

Why is weight control so important? After all, only a century ago being heavy was considered a sign of status and wealth. Well, since then we've learned what a spare tire portends for a man. Obesity—and particularly obesity around the middle, where men tend to carry fat—is associated with all sorts of health problems. Fat men often develop insulin resistance, which can lead to diabetes. They also are more likely to have high blood pressure and high cholesterol. (The latter may, at least in part, be the result of what men eat to get fat.) The net result is an increase in risk of heart disease. For men between thirty and forty-four years old, each body-mass index point (see below) above 21 increases the risk of heart attack by 10 percent; risk is increased less for older men but is still very large.

The good news is that losing weight and keeping it off is a lot easier than you and he probably think.

Does He Weigh What He Should?

Doctors used to rely on weight tables that told how much a person of each height should weigh. Lately, most prefer instead the body-mass index, or BMI. Your man's BMI should be between 19 and 25. While a BMI of 20 is good and 40 is very bad, don't take the difference between 24 and 26 too seriously. First of all, BMI can't tell muscle from fat. Men who build muscle readily may have a BMI higher than 25 without carrying too much fat. Also, because this formula is simplified, the BMI you calculate may be off by as much as 2. Calculate using the following steps:

1. Multiply body weight in pounds by .45. Example: 175 pounds × .45 = 78.75.

2. Multiply height in inches by .025. Example: 72 inches × .025 = 1.8.

3. Multiply the result of step 2 by itself. Example: 1.8 × 1.8 = 3.24.

4. Divide the answer from step 1 by the answer from step 3. Example: 78.75 ÷ 3.24 = 24.3.

Beyond Dieting

Compared to him, you probably already know a lot about weight loss, but you probably have also been exposed to more misleading and damaging diet myths than he has. Like many women, have you lost weight several times, only to gain it back? Have *your* pants been shrinking the past few years? Have you cut back on meals—maybe skipped breakfast—in an unsuccessful attempt to lessen the fabric strain around your thighs? Despite claims made by many diet books, products, and programs, the solution isn't starvation, magic pills, or totally eliminating a food. Before you can help your man, you first have to abandon the traditional notion of "diet."

Extreme or fad diets don't work. Oh, sure, people lose weight on crash diets. The problem is that they lose it over and over again. Fully 95 percent of people who diet regain all the weight within five years. Even worse, yo-yo dieting—repeatedly losing and gaining weight—works against your body's metabolism and may even increase the risk of heart disease.

The problem with weight-loss diets is that you can't sustain them. For example, you can lose weight on a high-protein, low-carbohydrate diet, but you can't eat that way for the rest of your life. When you go back to eating normally, the pounds reappear. In fact, you will put on weight even faster, thanks to a built-in survival mechanism. When you restrict calories, the body slows its resting metabolic rate, the rate at which you burn calories to fuel such activities as breathing, pumping blood, and digesting food. The body thinks it is facing starvation, so it wisely slows down and then needs less food to get by. When you start eating normally again, your body will burn the calories less efficiently, and you'll gain weight faster than ever. A drop in metabolism also causes a frustrating plateau midway through a diet. If you cut calories by 500 per day and lose five pounds, you'll have to cut calories even more to lose another five pounds.

I know a couple who is always in one of two phases: a diet that involves denying themselves good food and substituting "diet formulas," or overeating what they really want and gaining it all back.

Worst of all, a weight-loss diet reduces the body's ratio of fat to muscle. When there is insufficient food to maintain its tissues, your body sheds the ones that use the most energy (your muscles) before it gives up the ones that take less energy to maintain (your fat). You keep fat tissue and lose muscle tissue even if the pounds go down.

Magic Pills?

Wouldn't it be nice if we could just pop a pill, then keep on eating what we always have and get thin? Men love this sort of "silver bullet" approach to health. Unfortunately, even the new weight-loss medications have their down side. Most people do lose more weight when they take them, but most people also regain the weight when they stop. Some people experience side effects, including dry mouth, nausea, headache, and a rare but dangerous lung disease. Furthermore, the pills cost between $15 and $75 a month. Diet pills are for seriously overweight people and should supplement, not replace, eating better and exercising. If he can trim down without pills, he'll be much better off.

A Bit Less In, a Bit More Burned Off

If extreme or crash diets aren't the answer, what is? It's really quite simple: Subtract a few calories and add some activity. The best results are achieved by approaching fat loss from both directions: by eating carefully *and* exercising. When he burns more than he takes in, he'll start to lose body fat. To lose half a pound of body fat a week, which is a smart, sustainable goal, he needs a 1,750-calorie deficit. Just 250 fewer calories eaten, or 250 calories more burned off per day, will do the job—one uneaten fast-food hamburger or a half-hour brisk walk.

Although he doesn't need a big calorie deficit each day, if he has a slight calorie excess, he will gain weight over time. If a man eats half a gram of fat too much each day, he will put on nearly forty pounds between twenty and sixty. Considering that he'll eat more than eighteen tons of food during those forty years, the excess food is tiny—less than a tenth of 1 percent.

On the exercise side of the equation, each week he should put in three aerobic exercise sessions, each at least thirty minutes long, and two strength-training sessions. Exercise is important because it increases his metabolism, the rate at which his body burns food. For each pound of muscle put on through strength training, he'll burn 30 to 50 more calories a day, even on lazy days. Strength training also creates a pronounced "afterburn." After exercising, his metabolism stays high for some time; the length depends on the intensity of the exercise and the individual. Furthermore, exercise offsets the decline in metabolism that happens as he grows older. Without vigorous exercise, a man's internal flame gradually weakens. After a big meal, a sixty-year-old man burns 87 fewer calories than does a twenty-year-old man—unless the older guy exercises regularly to even the tab. A forty-eight-year-old triathlete friend of mine is proof positive of the relationship between exercise and eating: Watching how much he eats can be a distressing experience, but by the looks of him, he puts it to good use.

Not only does exercise increase the body's metabolism so that it burns more calories, but it also takes the weight off where it matters: at the belt line. A bulging waistline—a body with an "apple shape"—increases the risk of heart disease, high blood pressure, stroke, and diabetes. If his waist at its narrowest place is wider than his hips, that signals trouble. Fortunately, the first place aerobic exercise removes fat is the midsection. In a University of Washington study, older men who took up intense aerobic exercise lost 20 percent of their belt-line fat in six months, nearly twice as much as they lost from their arms or legs.

Watch Fats for Easy Calories

Most of the easy ways to cut 250 calories involve reducing the amount of fat in the diet. The reason is simple arithmetic: Each gram of fat contains 9 calories, while a gram of protein or carbohydrate contains only 4. To be low in fat, a food should have less than 30 percent of its calories from fat. Cutting fats also helps reduce artery-clogging cholesterol and has other health benefits (see the previous chapter).

Where to Find 250 Calories per Day That He Won't Miss

If he's exercising, the rest of the diet equation is pretty easy. Some simple techniques can shape up his diet and trim down his middle.

A good place to start is **breakfast.** Encourage him to eat it every day and have appealing, healthful foods on hand. Skipping meals lowers metabolism; not eating breakfast can cause him to burn 80 fewer calories per day. Perhaps even more important, a missed breakfast often leads to a 10:00 A.M. doughnut or lunchtime gluttony.

Taper meals through the day. In most American households the evening meal is the largest. That's exactly the opposite of what it should be. Try to make breakfast and lunch—which we follow with food-burning activity—the more substantial meals. Keep dinner lighter since we have less need for energy at night. Some nutritionists think that by merely eating more in the first half of the day than in the second half, many men will start shedding body fat.

Encourage him to **eat less more often.** Because eating boosts metabolism, doing it more often keeps metabolism higher. Instead of dividing his daily calories into two or three meals, he might enjoy five smaller meals a day. The mid-morning and mid-afternoon snacks can be relatively small; I like a hard-boiled egg without the yolk, a low-fat bran muffin, low-fat yogurt, and fruit. In the summer my wife and I cut up a bowl of fruit in the morning and take some along for snacks. Healthy snacks will help him stay revved up and will keep him from being so hungry that he overeats at mealtime.

Serve smaller portions. In many households food left on the plate is considered an insult to the chef or practically a mortal sin. To disarm clean-plate syndrome, dish up modest amounts. Use smaller plates so the meal doesn't look small, and try covering some of that area with garnish. It is better for him to ask for more than for him to eat more than he really wants simply because it's already on his plate.

Get fiber into his first course. Serve a salad before the main course arrives so he'll fill up on the healthful, low-calorie vegetables before the heavier stuff appears. (Put the dressing in a small cup next to the salad so he'll use less.) For breakfast, put out grapefruit, melon, or oatmeal before (or instead of) the bacon and eggs.

Show him how to **eat at a leisurely pace.** We live in a hurry-up world and tend to approach food at the same frenetic pace. Unfortunately, it takes time for our stomachs to tell our brains that we've had enough, so we eat too much.

Set the table and sit down together. If you eat slowly, he'll slow down to keep you company and eat less as a result.

Dining with friends is fun, but it can lead to overeating. In particular, he's more likely to eat dessert at social meals. This may be a hard habit to break, but you can set an example by **declining dessert yourself.** Instead, relax over a cappuccino made with skim milk. Another dessert option is fresh fruit. Every once in a while, order one dessert with two forks—very romantic.

Beware of reduced-fat prepared foods. Although skim or low-fat milk is a great choice, the current rage for "lite" foods has pitfalls. Although the fat reduction is often minor, people take the label as a license to eat twice as much. In general, if you avoid prepared foods, light or regular, and instead cook your own dishes from fresh ingredients, your meals will taste better, have less fat and more nutrients, and won't be nearly as salty. Assuming that you do the shopping, just keep those things out of the freezer. Also keep in mind that a prepared food can be free of cholesterol yet still contain fat. Bachelors are notorious suckers for the frozen-food section at the supermarket. When I'm at the grocery store, I often see them patrolling the freezers as if they're looking for Mom in shrink-wrap. They clearly buy according to slogans on the package, not the details on the nutrition label. With your coaching, your man will be wiser.

Disarm the potato-chip monster; **take a strategic approach to snacks.** Instead of waiting for him to rummage through the cupboard, put out a tray of vegetables with a low-fat dip and a bowl of pretzels.

Reduce fat slowly. We've all heard of a "sweet tooth"; I'm convinced that many people also have a "fat tooth." Reducing fat in his diet too quickly may well cause yearnings that lead to binges. We can get used to a lower-fat diet if we do it gradually.

One way to cut fat is to **eat vegetarian once a week.** That may sound like a radical prescription for your carnivorous guy, but in some entrees he'll hardly notice what's missing. Try meatless lasagna made with low-fat ricotta cheese; chili without the beef but bursting with garlic, cumin, and onion; homemade burritos smothered in salsa and filled with fat-free beans and low-fat cheese; or homemade pizza with vegetable toppings and low-fat mozzarella. Hey, he'll let you get away with it once a week.

Another way to lessen the presence of red meat is to **serve fish or seafood twice a week.** They are nutritional powerhouses, and most types are low in fat.

To round out a week of lower-fat eating, **put skinless chicken or (even better) turkey on the table twice a week.** Herbs and spices can compensate for the missing fat. Try rosemary, marjoram, sage, or garlic. You can cook fowl with its skin on to retain moistness, but remove it before serving because about four-fifths of the fat in chicken or turkey is in the skin. When skinless, both types of poultry are very low in fat and are excellent sources of protein.

You still have two days left in the week. Go ahead and serve him beef if that's what he craves. Trim the fat before cooking and use the leaner grades of hamburger.

Finally, **watch out for autumn.** For reasons that aren't entirely clear, we seem to lose our sense of fullness in the fall. A Georgia State University study found that people eat an average of 220 more calories a day as the sun drops lower in the sky. Be particularly watchful at that time of year and encourage him to exercise more in the pleasant, cool weather.

Of course, all these tips may not work if you're stuck with a man who won't cooperate. Some men seem bent on dietary self-destruction. I've known men who wouldn't cut down on the fatty snacks when their doctors *ordered* them to lose weight after a heart attack. Don't take the burden of his misbehavior on your shoulders. For a man like this, you'll only face frustration if you try to be the "food cop." Instead, ask for help from authority figures. A call from his doctor might set him straight, or you might enlist the help of a relative—an older brother is always good. For your own part, make it clear that you want him around a while longer. One of the best motivators is love. You're not feeding him celery to punish him!

Empty Calories

Among the ways to overindulge in calories, drinking alcoholic beverages is one of the easiest and most efficient. Booze contains almost nothing of use to the human body other than empty calories. One regular twelve-ounce beer delivers 140 calories; even a "light" beer has 95. No wonder a big gut got the nickname "beer belly." A six-ounce glass of table wine adds 120, and a shot (one-and-a-half ounces) of 80-proof liquor, 100 calories. It doesn't take much of any of these drinks to erase that 250-per-day calorie deficit he's been working on.

Tips for Eating on the Road

For many men, home isn't the danger zone when it comes to eating. Restaurants are. When others prepare his food, both of you lose control over ingredients and portion size. A restaurant's livelihood depends on making him a happy, sated customer, and the most dependable approach is lots of butter and big helpings of fried foods.

Since he's not as savvy about nutrition as you are, he's likely to be duped by restaurant fare that seems as if it should be healthy and is anything but. For example, most restaurant bran muffins contain little fiber and a load of fat. He's safer sticking with whole wheat toast. Granola is often made with lots of oil and nuts, so unless it has been specially designed to be low in fat, it's no more healthy than a sugary kids cereal. A bare bagel of modest size is a great morning starter. But have you noticed that bagels keep getting bigger and bigger? I'll bet he hasn't. A typical bagel these days packs about 300 calories—the same as five slices of toast—and I've seen some with 460 calories. A layer of cream cheese adds hundreds of fat-rich calories. He can even run into trouble if he orders that staple of diet plates: cottage cheese. Low-fat cottage cheese is a great source of protein and calcium, but the restaurant variety is often made with whole milk—which makes it creamy—and may get nearly half its calories from fat.

Ethnic restaurants can also be confusing territory for a man looking for a low-fat meal. Faced with familiar American fare, he can order baked or grilled chicken, sauce on the side. But is moo goo gai pan low-fat? You can help him out by sharing some basic ethnic cuisine guidelines.

The first rule of low-fat **Chinese** eating is to avoid fried foods such as egg rolls, fried wontons, fried rice, and sweet-and-sour dishes. He should also stay away from nut-based sauces. The notorious kung pao, for example, is based on fat-rich peanuts, and many other Chinese dishes include fatty cashews. Seafood choices, such as Szechuan shrimp, offer the lowest fat content. Whichever dish he chooses, suggest that he get the sauce on the side; I find that only half as much as usual provides full flavor. Also, do as the Chinese do and have a generous serving of steamed rice, which is low in fat and rich in carbohydrates.

The staples of the **Mexican** diet, rice and beans, are healthful ways to fuel a man. However, frying and the add-ons can gum up his works. First of all, say no to that basket of chips. It can fill his fat quota well before he sees an entree. Nachos combine fried chips *and* high-fat cheese. Seek restaurants that offer whole beans rather than refried ones, which are often cooked with lard to give them flavor and a smooth texture. Then point him toward the fajitas or a chicken burrito, two of the lower-fat options on the menu. Sour cream and guacamole can double the fat count of an otherwise healthful burrito; help him get in the habit of asking the cook to leave them off.

Italian food has been unduly maligned. True, many of the favorites— cheese-stuffed pastas such as ravioli, rich cream sauces such as Alfredo, and oil- and nut-based sauces such as pesto—are fearsome fat feasts. But there are many wonderful dishes that make Italian one of the most healthful cuisines. Pasta can be adorned with a variety of great low-fat sauces. The basic tomato sauce is called marinara, but he also ought to try primavera (with vegetables) or one based on mushrooms or wine. Seafood mixtures also make excellent choices. Look for shrimp, mussels, or clams in a tomato base. Be sure he fills up on crusty Italian bread before the main course arrives; it's good enough to eat without the butter or olive oil.

It's tempting to say he should give up **fast food** entirely, but let's be realistic. The best you can hope is to turn it from a staple into an occasional treat. With a few exceptions nothing on a fast-food menu is low in fat. Grilled or broiled chicken sandwiches may qualify, if ordered without the sauce, but breaded or fried chicken is little better than beef. It does help to order the regular-sized hamburgers or other sandwiches instead of the double cheese-burger with bacon or other souped-up items. French fries are a potato medium designed to absorb fat. Perhaps he can be persuaded to order the smaller size. Some fast-food restaurants offer a baked potato or a salad bar. A happy surprise at the fast-food order window is the milk shake. The offerings from the larger chains actually contain little milk, so their fat content is typically less than 20 percent. That chocolate shake he's been hankering for turns out to be a great place to start his next McMeal.

Food Is Still Love

While maintaining a healthy weight is very important, if you treat food as medicine, both you and your man will think of it in a negative way. Just as it's always been, food is love.

Eating should be a positive experience. Focus on wonderful things to eat rather than on what not to eat. Involve him in planning the day's meals. Explore new restaurants together. Show your love for each other by sharing delectable, heart-healthy meals.

9

Mr. Sandman

At night, do you and your man share seven hours of restful companionship, or do you share your sleep problems instead? When a couple sleeps together, each partner depends on the other to sleep well. If one has trouble falling asleep or awakens during the night, the tossing and turning can keep the other partner up, too. If one snores (and you know which one that'll be), he'll probably wake the other up.

Too little sleep or sleep that's too shallow because it's constantly disrupted is called sleep deprivation. Not only does it make a person tired and cranky the next day, but it can cause anxiety, poor job performance, and impairment of memory and concentration. Most dangerously, daytime sleepiness greatly increases the risk of accidents, including while driving. Inhibited deep sleep in older people—particularly men—can dramatically reduce production of growth hormone, which decreases the amount of muscle and increases the accumulation of fat. Sleep apnea, in which breathing actually stops for at least ten seconds during snoring, has been linked to a higher risk of cardiovascular problems. Just how serious is sleep loss? Laboratory rats deprived of sleep die within about two and a half weeks.

If sleep is elusive at your house, it's time to look for solutions. For successful sleep, *both* of you have to understand your sleep patterns, develop good sleep habits, and seek treatment for any sleep disorder.

Dancing in Circadian Rhythm

If you or your partner has trouble falling or staying asleep (called insomnia) or is sleepy in the morning, the first step is to get back in tune with your natural sleep rhythm, your "circadian rhythm." Humans have biological clocks that make us sleepy at regular intervals even if we haven't been active. (Sleep isn't simply what happens when the burdens of the day have worn us out.) The human circadian rhythm insists we get some shut-eye between one and four in the morning. It also urges us to nap between one and four in the afternoon, a time when traffic accidents are particularly common. (My patients who are truck drivers usually know to watch out for the wee morning hours, but few know about the afternoon dip.) Our sleep cycles are strongly influenced by the pattern of light and dark each twenty-four hours.

Too often we ignore the message that it's time to sleep. While humans need just as much sleep as ever, the average American gets by on one-and-a-half to two hours less sleep per night than did his or her grandparents at the turn of the century. What's more, we often don't follow the natural cycle of dark and light. Between 15 and 20 percent of Americans now work a schedule other than the day shift. Even those of us lucky enough to have day jobs don't sleep from sunset to sunrise. More likely we go to bed hours after dark and, in summer at least, rise well after the sun has come up. Instead of sleeping we watch TV, surf the net, get caught up on household chores, shop, or work into the night. Because we're out of sync with our natural sleep cycles, we then have trouble falling and staying asleep.

To get in rhythm, start by setting a wake-up time that will allow you and your partner to get to work or meet other responsibilities in the morning. Then work backward to find your new bedtime. Build in the amount of sleep you feel you need each night, probably between seven and nine hours. Once you've set the rise time, stick with it. Don't sleep in on weekends or holidays, which you've probably been doing to try to make up for lost sleep. As much as possible follow your bedtime schedule every day. At first you may not be able to fall asleep right away. Gradually your internal clocks will adjust to the regular wake-up time, allowing you to get to sleep earlier. Regularity is a fundamental part of healthful sleep habits.

If you have trouble shifting your sleep time, you can alter the times you feel wakeful and get sleepy through exposure to bright light at certain times of day. If your bedmate can't shut down in the evening, urge him to wake at the right time in the morning (even though he doesn't want to) and go outside in the bright sun (artificial light boxes are also available). Within about a week his circadian rhythm will begin to shift backward, allowing him to get to sleep earlier.

Some sleep specialists also use a technique called chronotherapy to alter a patient's sleep cycle. A person whose problem is a late bedtime just goes to sleep later and later, shifting his bedtime *forward* a few hours per day until bedtime has been shifted all the way around the clock to the proper time. The fact that such a technique works shows the power of our biological clock.

Whatever method you and your partner use to set a better sleep cycle, adjust your other activities to fit the new schedule. You may have to eat dinner earlier, give up on late-night talk shows, or even switch off the phone at 9:00. The rest of your habits must fit your new sleep pattern, or it won't stick.

You may find that your natural sleep rhythms are different from your partner's. There actually are morning people and night people, and for some reason they usually pair up. You may have to make peace with different schedules. Though I know I sleep better with my wife than when I have to travel alone, our sleep rhythms are different, and we had to figure out how to adapt to each other's cycles. I typically fall asleep an hour or two before she does in the evening, and I'm out of bed an hour or two before her in the morning. For us that means she gets an hour or so of peace and quiet at night, and I enjoy the stillness of the house first thing in the morning. Although our patterns aren't the same, each of us gets a good night's sleep and awakens refreshed and ready to start a new day.

Create a Sleepy Environment

If at all possible, make your bedroom a place exclusively for sleep. Try to put your home office, exercise machine, and computer in other parts of the house. I know the TV has become a fixture in the American bedroom, but for many people the stimulation gets in the way of a sound snooze. Sleep is a subtle thing, and the smallest tension can disrupt it.

Make sure that your sleeping environment is as comfortable as possible. First and foremost, that means a comfortable bed. If yours is old or has never really been comfortable, go shopping. Experiment with pillows—not only the type of stuffing but also the shape, size, and number. The final component is all-cotton sheets in summer and flannel sheets in winter. Sure they wrinkle, but they're far more comfortable against the skin than synthetics. Each day he wears those sheets at least as long as he wears a shirt at work.

The temperature in the bedroom also has to be right. Most of us sleep best with the room a bit cool. During sleep, body temperature drops, and for most people it's helpful if the air temperature does, too. Sweating is not conducive to a good night's sleep. A quiet ceiling fan set on its lowest speed helps many couples stay comfortable at night. Down comforters can help couples with different ideal temperatures because the filling can be shifted over the chilly

Buying a Bed for Two

• Do you or your mate toss and turn trying to find a comfortable position?

• Do you roll toward each other during the night? (It's only romantic if you *mean* to.)

• If either of you sleeps on your front, is your back sore in the morning?

• Do you sleep better if you put the mattress on the floor for a few nights?

If you or your guy answers "yes" to any of these questions, you need a new bed that conforms to your shape and the way you sleep. The only way to pick the right one is to test-drive some. Don't be shy. Spend no less than ten minutes lying on a prospective bed in each position that you like to sleep in. You should sense that your weight is being supported evenly by as much of your body as possible. Women tend to have problems with concentrated pressure on the hips, and men on their shoulders. If either of you senses that you're sagging between your hips and shoulders, move on to another mattress. After spending some time in the test position, either you'll still be comfortable or you'll be getting hints that a full night on that bed would include a lot of tossing and turning.

Most people sleep best on a medium-firm mattress that has a medium-soft top layer. You may find that you and your partner need different degrees of firmness. After all, you *are* shaped somewhat differently. That doesn't mean you must have separate beds. One side of the bed can be stiffened by adding a layer of plywood between the mattress and box spring or softened on top by adding a layer of foam rubber beneath the mattress pad. Experiment until you're both happy.

Also consider the size of the mattress. A double bed is fine for some couples, but others need more room so they don't kick or bump each other during the night.

person. Finally, humidity needs to be maintained in the comfort range, 40 to 60 percent.

Because periods of light and dark modulate our circadian rhythm, it's important that the bedroom be very, or even completely, dark. If you live in a metropolitan or suburban area, you probably need curtains or blinds. If possible, though, leave windows that face the rising sun uncovered. Sunlight in the bedroom in the morning helps make rising easier and sets the right mood for the day.

What if your spouse's sleep pattern—like mine—is offset from yours by an hour or so? Leaving a light on in the evening for reading can make it harder for your partner to get to sleep and may hold up his progression to deep sleep. If so, he needs a blindfold. Available in pharmacies and department stores, the black pad with an elastic band slips over his head and creates a soothing cocoon of complete darkness.

Just as too much light can delay and disturb sleep, so can noise. His snoring, for example, can wreak havoc on your night's rest. We'll discuss that obvious form of noise in a few pages, but for the moment think about other noises. Do you start the dishwasher just before going to bed? Is the kitchen close enough to your bedroom that you can hear the plates clinking against each other? Even if the noise doesn't prevent the two of you from getting to sleep or wake you up, it will affect the quality of your sleep. Even while sleeping, our ears and nervous systems register sounds, reducing the depth of sleep. Tonight when you go to bed, concentrate on what you hear. Tomorrow, work on ways to reduce the noise in your sleeping environment even if it means wearing earplugs to bed.

Other Ways to Improve Sleep

Send him out for a workout. I know I'm beginning to sound like a broken record, recommending exercise over and over, but exercise is good for sleep, too. Not only does it alleviate physical and mental stress that can keep him awake, but by raising the body's temperature for a few hours, it enhances the drop to the lower temperature at night. Men who exercise fall asleep more quickly, sleep up to an hour longer, and enjoy a third more deep sleep. To gain the most from the drop in temperature, he needs to exercise in the late afternoon or early evening. One guy I know shifted his lunch hour to 3:00 in the afternoon so he could work out during a time when he otherwise would be inclined to nap. He was surprised to find that he slept much better at night. If you haven't yet convinced your spouse to exercise, let alone do it in the mid-afternoon, go for a walk with him after an early dinner. He should avoid exercising right before bed, though, because it's too stimulating.

He should also **consider what he's eating** right before going to bed.

Digestion does make one drowsy, but if you stuff yourself, the discomfort gets in the way of sound sleep. On the other hand, going to bed hungry can lead to a middle-of-the-night snack. (People on very-low-calorie diets often have trouble sleeping through the night.)

Some people find that a light snack about thirty minutes before bedtime helps them get to sleep. Sleep specialists argue about whether the snack should be protein, carbohydrate, or some combination. If you or your partner falls into the snack-before-bed crowd, you probably already have a good idea about what works best. Avoid fatty foods packed with calories and food laced with sugar that will work on your teeth all night.

If your man is over fifty, the odds are even that his prostate is enlarged to some degree. That may cause one or more bathroom breaks during the night, which can be very disturbing to sleep. Although copious amounts of water are great for the prostate during the day, he should **stop drinking water within two hours of bedtime.** In addition, if he takes diuretics, he should do so in the morning, not at nighttime. It almost goes without saying that alcohol and caffeine are strict no-nos for guys on the go. But he'll also benefit from spending some time making sure he voids completely before going to bed. Often there's more urine to be released if he takes the time and relaxes fully. (And if he hasn't seen his doctor about that prostate, he should in any case.)

He should not have that nightcap. Alcohol is very likely to disturb sleep. A nightcap may help him doze off and even keep him asleep for the first half of the night, but then he'll probably wake up and sleep only fitfully for the rest of the night. Furthermore, alcohol affects sleep quality even when it's consumed hours before bedtime. During the first half of the night, he will experience much less REM sleep. (Rapid Eye Movement sleep is the time when we dream, which is essential for restorative sleep. It's also the time when men experience nocturnal erections—three to five of them per night, lasting as long as forty minutes each, and recharging his sexual batteries.) Then, after he wakes in the middle of the night, he'll get little but REM sleep—leaving out the other important sleep phases. Perhaps most troubling of all, depending on alcohol to get to sleep is a common step toward alcoholism.

Most people know better than to drink coffee after dinner, but he should also **prevent caffeine from sneaking into his late-night life** in other forms. Tea contains much less of the stimulant per cup, but if he consumes three or four cups, he'll be counting sheep for hours. Likewise, most sodas, a staple of the American diet, contain caffeine. Some of the clear ones, such as Mountain Dew and Surge, contains lots. Is he considering chocolate cake for dessert? There's caffeine in chocolate. Many of the heavily advertised drugstore pain relievers that promise to quell a headache contain a significant jolt of caffeine.

You probably already know most of the reasons he should **give up tobacco,** but here's another one: Smoking can be very disruptive to sleep. Nicotine is a powerful and addictive stimulant. Smoking may make it harder to get to sleep, and a smoker is likely to wake up repeatedly during the night as the body insists on another puff. In the next chapter I'll talk more about how to quit smoking, but be aware that if your partner uses the nicotine patch to help him quit, a sixteen-hour patch that's removed at night is less likely to disrupt his sleep.

It helps to **prepare mentally for sleep.** Few of us would enjoy leaping from bed and immediately performing calculus or running a mile. Each of us has a morning ritual—shower, shave, brush teeth, the paper, etc.—that prepares our minds for the activities of the day. We don't burst upon the day each morning, so there's no reason to think that we should go in the other direction—from maximum activity to sleep—in minutes. We need an evening ritual to help us gradually gear down for bedtime. Between thirty and sixty minutes before bedtime, abandon everyday business. No more work on that report that is due soon, no more paying the bills, no more balancing the checkbook. It's time to begin slowing down for sleep. A little quiet music may set the mood for putting minor things in order. Your partner could make sure the dog is properly bedded down or check to be sure the outside lights are on and the doors are closed and locked. He could set the table for tomorrow's breakfast or check on the children. The evening ritual must not be stressful; it should involve simple, methodical tasks which give a sense that things are in order. To be a ritual it must be done *every* night. Finish the ritual with washing your face and brushing your teeth—or even taking a warm bath together. Feeling clean is relaxing, too. When you can do these little things automatically every evening without even being very aware of them, you will have established behaviors that tell your brain that sleep time is coming.

Just as important as developing a good evening ritual is avoiding a bad one. The most common sleep-disruptive behavior among my male friends is napping in front of the TV in the easy chair before getting up to get ready for bed. When a guy dozes off before he's actually in bed, it can completely confuse his sleep clock. Quite often he'll be wide awake by the time he can get tucked in. Arrange the evening so that you maintain activity until it's time for the get-sleepy ritual. Hobbies—from woodworking to car restoration—are

Drugs That Can Affect Sleep

If he's having sleep problems, the culprit may be a medication he's taking. Encourage him to ask his doctor or pharmacist whether the medication can affect sleep. Far too many people assume that they just have to live with the side effects of their medications. In fact, individual reactions to medications are almost as diverse as our responses to music. If one medication is keeping him awake at night, there's an excellent chance that switching to another that's equally effective will let him rest well. Prescriptions aren't commandments; doctors should listen attentively to reports of side effects and be willing to suggest alternatives. These medications are among those that can affect sleep:

Amphetamines (occasionally prescribed for weight loss)

Antianxiety medications (when benzodiazepines, such as Xanax, are discontinued)

Antidepressants (selective seratonin reuptake inhibitors, such as Prozac, and monoamine oxidase inhibitors, such as Nardil)

Appetite suppressants (such as Adipex-P and Redux)

Blood pressure medications (some but not all; check with your doctor or pharmacist)

Caffeine (present in many headache preparations)

Cholesterol-lowering agents

Corticosteroids (such as prednisone)

Levodopa (for treatment of Parkinson's disease)

Methysergide (prescribed for severe vascular headaches)

Nicotine

Theophylline (for asthma)

Thyroid-replacement hormone (when dosage is too high)

helpful because they can be picked up and set aside easily on a nightly basis, and completion is generally weeks or months down the line. Just be sure he stops on schedule and begins that evening ritual.

Many people have swollen feet and legs at the end of the day. It's hard to get to sleep with throbbing legs. If this troubles him, **suggest that he put his feet up for an hour or two before bedtime.**

Develop a plan for dealing with mid-night wake-ups. One of the most common sleep problems among adults is waking up at 1:00 or 2:00 and not being able to get back to sleep. The world can take on an ominous cast at 3:00 A.M. Some of the techniques I've mentioned previously should help reduce the frequency of mid-night sleeplessness, but you should still prepare for the possibility. If either of you is prone to waking up and thinking about things you have to do the next day, put a pencil and paper by the bed and write those things down when they come to mind. Thoughts that are recorded on paper are easier to put out of mind. Some people are helped by writing down their worries, too. When they're reviewed in the light of day, they usually seem pretty silly, which helps condition us to worry less at night.

A basic principle of mid-night sleeplessness is not to give up too quickly. Once you turn the light on, you're going to be awake for a while. (Remember the messages that light sends to your biological clock?) On the other hand, there's no sense battling grimly to get back to sleep. At some point you need to admit you're awake and restart the ritual toward sleep. Have that blindfold close at hand for your partner and switch on the light. Reading for a little while may help, as may a light snack. Just checking on the children or testing the doors to see that they really are locked can help you relax and get back to sleep. You might say that sleep is a state of mind that requires a state of mind to get there.

Sawing Logs

After fifty, most men snore, and about a third of younger guys snore, too. You are less than half as likely to be a noisy sleeper. Do you *know* beyond a doubt that he snores—though he maintains that he doesn't? Join the crowd. About three times as many women say their mates snore as there are men who will admit to it. You're also in good company if you are irritated about it. Women name snoring as the number one bedroom annoyance (men put it behind such bothers as hogging the covers and cold feet).

Unfortunately, cartoon characters have perpetuated the myth that snoring is a sign of deep sleep. Nothing could be further from the truth. People snore because their airway becomes constricted when they breathe, causing flesh in their throat to vibrate. *You are not doing him any favors by suffering through his snoring or grudgingly moving to another room.* Because snoring interferes with breathing, it can lower oxygen levels in the blood, rousing the sleeper from time to time. Sleep apnea takes this to the extreme, endangering his health. What's more, the noise bothers not only you but also him, reducing the amount of restorative REM sleep he gets each night. Snoring is not natural. It's also not inevitable—there are many possible solutions.

- **Help him lose weight.** Fat deposits in his throat make the airway smaller for breathing, increasing the likelihood that he will snore. Two-thirds of people with sleep apnea are obese.

- **Ask him to sleep on his side.** Most men snore on their backs and make little noise on their sides or stomachs. When he's on his back, his jaw can slip backward, collapsing his throat and causing snoring. Longer, firmer pillows can help him sleep on his side since they will support his head. As a last resort, sew a tennis ball into the back of his nightshirt so he'll be dissuaded from rolling onto his back.

- **Help him substitute sparkling water for beer.** Not only does alcohol disrupt sleep cycles, but it also relaxes muscles in the neck, collapsing his airway. Studies have shown that drinkers are much more prone to apnea, in part because the airway is smaller but also because alcohol suppresses breathing function by as much as half. Many men without sleep apnea develop it as soon as they drink.

- **Convince him to stop smoking.** (Here we go again.) Besides disrupting sleep, smoking increases nasal congestion, leading to mouth breathing and you know what. Furthermore, smoking contributes to the diseases to which men with sleep apnea are prone: high blood pressure, stroke, and heart disease.

- **Buy him nasal strips.** Those pieces of tape you see on athletes' noses can also help him breathe easier, reducing the likelihood of snoring. Today they're even marketed as sleep aids, and you should be able to find them at your local pharmacy.

- **Send him to the dentist.** The dentist or orthodontist can fit him with a device that restrains his tongue from slipping backward in his throat or prevents his jaw from moving backward, either of which can restrict the airway. This is particularly effective for men who just won't sleep in any position except on their back.

- **Make an appointment for him at a sleep center.** For men with diagnosed sleep apnea, an approach called nasal continuous positive airway pressure (CPAP) can be a great help. A mask fits tightly around the nose and a pump delivers air into the nasal passage, creating positive air pressure. CPAP improves sleep and nearly eliminates the symptoms of apnea (elevated blood pressure and irregular heartbeat) within a few days.

Medical Solutions for Sleep Problems

Although there's a lot you can do to help keep the peace in the bedroom, you don't have to work alone to find solutions. At long last sleep is being recognized as an important medical specialty, and doctors who specialize in it can be found in nearly all metropolitan areas and many smaller communities. Many universities also have sleep clinics and research centers.

Most sleep therapists will work with you on many of the techniques I've discussed here. They can also provide other, more advanced behavioral approaches, including stimulus control therapy, sleep restriction therapy, relaxation therapies, and cognitive therapy. Medication may also play a role. Usually a combination of medication and behavioral treatment works best. More than two-thirds of people who see a sleep specialist are sleeping much better two weeks later and are able to discontinue the medication. Besides insomnia, snoring, and sleep apnea, there are also dozens of other sleep

What About Pills?

Whether they're prescribed by a doctor or bought off the shelves of a drugstore, sleeping pills are only a temporary solution to sleep problems. Still, don't assume that he shouldn't be taking one. For many people just knowing that they are on the night stand if needed helps them relax and slip away. When sleeping pills are used in conjunction with behavioral treatments administered by sleep specialists, their track record is very good. However, self-administered, over-the-counter medicines (usually antihistamines) don't work as well. Most people suffer some degree of drug "hangover" from the OTC preparations, and effectiveness isn't well established.

The "natural drug" Melatonin hasn't turned out to be a panacea for sleeplessness. It may help some people drop off, but it has the opposite effect on others. Few people sleep better through the night. Melatonin has helped people suffering from jet lag because it can help readjust the circadian rhythm. But even for that use, it's difficult to determine how much is needed or to find dosages that are carefully controlled. (Most health food store preparations contain way too much.)

If he's going to take pills, he should see a doctor who specializes in sleep disorders and get the best.

disorders, and a sleep specialist can identify underlying problems and treat them.

Insomnia is so often a part of depression that it's a good idea to consider the list of signs of depression in chapter 12 and urge him to see his doctor if you see a pattern.

If bedtime continues to be anything but restful for you, please seek a specialist. Now you know how important sleep is to your well-being and your man's. Think of it this way: We can get along much longer without food or water than we can without sleep. Only breathing is more important, and with some sleep problems even that may be a problem. Sleep is fundamental to good health. Be sure you both get yours.

10

Risky Business

Why does he insist on taking chances? What compels him to drive too fast, smoke, play dangerous sports, or drink too much? No one knows for sure whether the culprit is his genes, his hormones, or the expectations and examples of other males. Although aggression has often been linked to testosterone, there's no link between an individual man's hormone levels and either his aggressiveness or the frequency of his risky behavior. (While football players rank high on testosterone, actors' levels are higher!) In part, the behavior may be learned since boys are encouraged to take risks and constantly see older men doing it.

Whatever the reason, most men are risk takers to some degree, and you'll only cause yourself misery if you try to tame yours. However, you can help him approach risks with an attitude of care rather than devil-may-care. The former is the intelligent man's approach; the latter is just plain stupid. You can tell him the facts about risks so he can decide which ones are worth taking. You can also help him approach risky activities as safely as possible.

It's one thing to put himself at risk and another to put you or your family at risk. If his risk-taking has crossed this line, you should definitely tell him how you feel about it. You have every right to insist that he drive carefully when you or the children are in the car. If he refuses to model safe behavior for your children by wearing a bicycle helmet, he deserves your scorn. If he continues to smoke, it shouldn't be inside your home. If his behavior is especially dangerous and he won't change, take steps to protect yourself and others.

Running on Empty

Almost all men see themselves as skilled drivers, but the statistics tell a different story. In 1994, 38,200 men were involved in fatal motor vehicle accidents, compared to only 14,600 women. Men are twice as likely as women to drink and drive, and they're less likely to wear seat belts. (Before you puff up too much with pride—women are more likely than men to be involved in fender benders, although by only a small margin.)

Paradoxically, while men take pride in their vehicles' appearance and attend to the mechanicals more faithfully than they take care of their own bodies, they wreck their cars far more often than women do. The reason is that men care about their cars so much that their egos get caught up in what they drive and how they drive it. Both the guy who drives a 350-horsepower sports cars at twenty miles per hour over the limit and the guy who drives a fifty-year-old pickup truck at twenty miles per hour under the limit are making personal statements that can lead them to exercise bad judgment.

Before a man can become a safe driver, he must disconnect his ego from his auto. Being passed by another driver must stop being a challenge. The car can no longer be a weapon. He must learn to think of driving as something he does to arrive at another location with minimum fuss and the least risk to man, beast, and bodywork.

Driving efficiently and wisely takes tremendous skill—far more than is taught in high school driver's education or than can be gained by simple experience. If your guy thinks he's a potential Richard Petty, buy him a driving school session for his birthday. Professional driving schools teach not only lifesaving car-control skills but also safety and humility. Because most such schools cater both to the everyday driver and to racers, safety is fundamental. Being around professional drivers dispels any doubts about whether safety belts are a good idea. And the elite skills exhibited by instructors quickly give the average guy some perspective on his own skill level. Most schools offer programs called "defensive driving" or "car control." The classes focus on the interplay between the physics of driving and the actions of the driver. They are oriented toward safe, skillful street driving. Some examples of schools include the Bob Bondurant School of High Performance Driving (800-842-7223) and Car Guys Decisive Driving Program (800-800-GUYS). Check your local yellow pages.

What if he wants a motorcycle? Yes, they are more dangerous than cars. But even if you could get away with saying no, would it affect your relationship? Will an appeal to his responsibility to family make the difference? Probably not. As with cars, your best bet is to help him ride as safely as possible. Encourage him to take the time and money to get all the training he can and to buy all the protective equipment (full-face helmet, protective boots, leather or other heavy jacket). The numbers are simple: Helmets reduce motorcycling fatalities by 30 percent. Once he's as safe as he can be, try to understand that he's enjoying himself to the fullest, and remember that he'll come home happy.

Accident Prone

Men have not only more car accidents but other kinds of accidents as well. They're seven times more likely than women to die in a firearm accident, five times more likely to drown, two and a half times more likely to be poisoned, and 50 percent more likely to die of burns. Accidents are the third leading cause of death in men, claiming almost sixty-thousand lives each year (for women, they're fifth).

You can't and shouldn't have to protect him from everything out there that bites. He's not a child. But there are easy, even fun, ways that can keep all of you further from such harm. Activities that are approached in a rational and well-prepared way become much less risky.

If you are a family of boaters, be sure that everyone learns to swim well, wears life jackets, and takes a boating-safety course from the Coast Guard Reserve or the Power Squadron. A local boat dealer should be able to give you contact numbers for members of these organizations. Classes are scheduled regularly in nearly all parts of the United States, and the lessons follow nationwide standards. They're lots of fun to take as a couple.

If there are firearms in your house, everyone of age should be trained in their use. Accidental firearm deaths are increasing most rapidly among young males, age ten to seventeen; since 1979 bullets have killed more children than members of the military. I hope your man chooses to steer clear of guns, but whether or not he does, he should understand how they work so that any he encounters don't work at the wrong time. Hunter-safety classes are offered regularly by state fish and wildlife agencies, and many local shooting clubs offer introductory classes. A phone call to a sporting goods store should turn up leads.

Still, the safest gun is no gun. You may not get far trying to talk him out of his collection, but you can insist on trigger locks. They're the surest way to secure guns in the home; they cost less than $10, prevent firing, and make firearms less attractive to thieves. If there are children (or visiting grand-children) in your home, reduce the risk of injury and death by keeping guns unloaded (with the trigger lock on) and stored in a locked cabinet or drawer.

Make sure the key is available only to responsible adults because children who know where the guns are kept may be tempted to show them off to their friends. Store ammunition in a separate locked cabinet. There have been many sad cases of young children finding guns their parents considered well hidden and accidentally shooting themselves, their siblings, or friends. Don't take a chance.

The risks associated with having guns in the home increase if any member of your household is depressed, has talked about suicide, is a troubled teenager, is violent toward others, abuses alcohol or other drugs, or has Alzheimer's disease. Talk over any concerns with your partner or your doctor.

Drinking Problems

Men who drink lightly appear to enjoy some health benefits. A five-ounce glass of wine, a beer, or a 1.5-ounce 80-proof cocktail (all containing roughly the same amount of alcohol) four or five days a week may reduce heart disease risk by as much as 40 percent. Once the intake is more than one a day (one every other day for women), benefits rapidly disappear. For men who take two or more drinks per day, death rates are 63 percent higher than for nondrinkers.

Many signs of a drinking problem are obvious, but others are subtle. Your man may be suffering from alcohol dependency if any one of the following statements is true. Does he:
- drink in the morning?
- lose his temper readily?
- lose coordination and stumble or fall?
- find it hard to relax or get to sleep without a drink?
- get sick while drinking?
- end up late for work because of a hangover?
- drive after drinking?
- frequently drink alone?
- become irritated when someone complains about his drinking?
- seem more argumentative when drinking?
- sometimes try to cut down but then relapses?

If he denies that he has a drinking problem, it will be very difficult to help him. First he must want to quit, and then he will probably need professional help. If he doesn't respond to gentle suggestions, ask your doctor for the names of specialists who treat alcohol dependency. Initially they can help you cope with the problem, and eventually they may be able to help him. Many hospitals and mental health centers also have programs. Another good resource is Alcoholics Anonymous, which organizes support groups for both alcoholics and the relatives of alcoholics, and can offer many tips to help you get through this troubling time.

It's important for both of you to remember that his drinking does not mean that either of you is a bad or inadequate person. He doesn't drink because you drive him to it, and he doesn't drink because he's a failure. Alcohol dependency is a medical problem that can be treated and cured.

Tobacco

About 42 percent of all male cancers are attributable to tobacco. One cigarette reduces his life span by twelve minutes, more time than it takes to smoke it.

If such statistics don't impress him, maybe the sexual forecast will. Men who smoke a pack a day for twenty years are 72 percent more likely than nonsmokers to develop impotence because of blocked arteries. About 70 percent of men with erection problems are smokers. Even before things stop working, a smoking man is less fertile. His semen will have lower sperm density, total count, and motility (activity). Appeal to his vanity, too. Smokers develop facial wrinkles sooner, turn gray prematurely, and may even be at greater risk of baldness.

It's a myth that a pipe, cigars, or oral tobacco are safe alternatives. All three can lead to oral cancers—about thirty thousand per year in the United States, of which nearly one-third are fatal. One type of oral cancer is so closely linked to tobacco that only 3.4 percent of those who develop it aren't tobacco users. Pipes and cigars also deliver plenty of nicotine. Guys who puff on these supposedly benign forms of tobacco are still three times more likely than nonsmokers to develop heart disease.

Of equal concern is what his smoking is doing to you and your family. Children whose parents smoke have far more respiratory illnesses, including coughs, colds, ear infections, pneumonia, and bronchitis. If they have asthma, the secondhand smoke worsens it and may trigger attacks. Later in life, people exposed to passive smoke as children will have a greater risk of heart problems and cancer. Secondhand smoke is particularly dangerous to infants and young children. If you are pregnant, passive smoke you breathe will enter the fetus.

Here again, pipes and cigars are not benign. In fact, one stogie launches about three times as many particles into the air as a cigarette and thirty times as much poisonous carbon monoxide.

The good news is that there's an excellent chance that your man really would like to quit smoking—70 percent of smokers say they wish they could. What's more, there's lots of help now to free him from the habit. If your man wants to quit smoking, encourage him to seek professional assistance. Even though nicotine patches and gum are now available without prescription, people who use them on their own are less likely to succeed. That's because smoking is both physically and psychologically addictive. Consider that smoking a pack a day involves repeating the same motions sixty thousand times a year. Nicotine gum or patches can help with the physical side, but to quit he needs to break his mental habits, too. People who use patches or gum and receive low-intensity counseling are twice as likely to stay off tobacco as those who try to quit solo. Of the two nicotine replacement approaches, patches are somewhat more successful than gum.

Once he decides to quit, he'll have to decide whether to reduce his smoking gradually or go cold turkey. Unless he's already a light smoker, his odds will be better if he cuts back before quitting. This plan minimizes withdrawal symptoms when the big day comes. During the first weeks he'll be less likely to feel depressed, anxious, or hungry, and he'll sleep better.

How to Smoke Less

For most smokers cutting down on the habit is the best preparation for giving it up entirely. Some or all of the following tips may help a loved one begin to loosen nicotine's grip.

- Keep cigarettes in only one place, and smoke only in that place.
- Switch brands to one that's less appealing.
- Smoke only the first half of each cigarette.
- Inhale only every other cigarette.
- Set a daily cigarette quota and keep a record.
- Postpone cigarettes from normal smoking times.
- Buy only by the pack, never by the carton.
- Wrap the cigarette pack in paper and close it with a rubber band. Unwrap and rewrap for each cigarette.
- Increase exercise. Cutting down on cigarettes will improve lung function, demonstrating a benefit of stopping.
- Smoke in uncomfortable places, such as outdoors in winter.
- Don't do anything else while smoking; think just about smoking.

When it comes time to quit, it's vital that he cut the string completely. The best chance of success is to stay completely smoke free for two weeks. Of those who slip during those two weeks, 90 percent end up smoking as much as they did previously.

To help break tobacco's grip, look for ways to eliminate its influence on his life. He should get rid of all cigarettes and cigarette lighters—not just by putting them in the trash but by actually destroying them. Then either throw away or wash and put away (in a deep cupboard) all the ashtrays. Make a dental appointment for him to get his teeth cleaned; without cigarettes he'll enjoy having his teeth stay that way.

One of the most difficult hurdles for long-term smokers is surviving the times when cigarettes were a daily habit: the smoke with the first cup of coffee in the morning, at morning work break, or even after sex. To get through these periods it helps to either completely change the activity or substitute a more healthful habit. If he's been having a smoke while making the morning coffee, maybe you can stand in for a while and bring him a cup in bed. At break time, instead of smoking with his coworkers, he might take a walk with some other colleagues. After sex, sips of water do more for afterglow than nicotine. Finally, suggest that he make a list of the reasons that he's quitting—including calculating just how much money he's saving—and read it at difficult times.

It takes roughly three weeks for the physical withdrawal symptoms from nicotine to disappear completely. That's why those first weeks are so important. However, the psychological urge to smoke can hang around for years. I know people who still dream about having a cigarette a decade after their last one. Nicotine addiction is powerful, but it's not unbeatable. Almost 40 million fewer Americans smoke now than did thirty years ago. Those who quit—myself included—and those who never took it up will enjoy a longer, more energetic life for it.

If he quits, make him feel great! Admire his improved physical stamina at the gym. Tell him to do something fun with all the money he is saving. Tell him how much you love his sweet kisses.

Sun Worship

A suntan is not a healthy golden glow. Sun exposure causes wrinkles and skin cancers, the most rapidly growing category of malignancies: 732,000 new cases a year, increasing at a rate of 100,000 every two years.

There's a lot of misunderstanding about how to reduce risk. Make sure your man knows the following:

• **Sunscreen helps, but it's not a total solution.** A lotion rated at least 15 and formulated to screen out both UVA and UVB radiation reduces the risk of some skin cancers, but it may not fully protect against the most deadly form, malignant melanoma. Also, sunscreen protects you for only a certain number of hours, no matter how high the rating. Long-sleeved, dark, tightly woven clothing and a hat with a brim complete the armaments. Also, it's smart to stay out of the direct sun at midday.

• **Dark skin doesn't necessarily protect him.** Fair-skinned, blue-eyed people are at greatest risk, but black men still get skin cancer—at one-tenth the rate, but who wants to be part of that tenth?

• **Skin cancer doesn't necessarily develop on the part of the skin exposed to the sun.** In men, malignant melanomas are usually found on the shoulders or hips. (Women most commonly get them on the lower legs or trunk.)

• **Tanning parlors are no safer**—and may be more dangerous—than natural sunlight.

A fondness for suntans is deeply embedded in our culture, but you can help pry it out. Don't compliment him on how good he looks tanned; do show a preference for his natural, unbaked skin tone. Subdue your own urge for more pigment—no small matter for many women. Your advantage is that you're much less likely to get sunburned out of stupidity. He may need to be reminded to put on the sunscreen, but you only have to remind yourself what's at stake.

Extreme Games

Men and sports are practically inseparable. Some men are satisfied with watching, but others want to be in the thick of it. Frequently, sports involve physical risk.

Many women are puzzled as to why we want to do something for fun that holds the potential for pain. It's not that we want to get hurt. We like to face the *possibility* of getting hurt and get away with it. It's not a death wish but a wish to thumb our noses at death. This may be stupid, but it's fundamental to the male psyche.

On the positive side, sports can motivate him to get in shape. For example, one of my patients is a sixty-year-old triathlete, a sport most people would consider extreme, particularly for a guy in his seventh decade. His conditioning stood him well, though, when he got prostate cancer. He withstood surgery like a man twenty years younger, and within three months he was competing again. His top-notch physical condition certainly helped. He also had incredible willpower and a spouse who supported him wholeheartedly.

If you are worried about his athletic endeavors, consider that they may not be nearly as dangerous as they seem. For example, scuba divers are fond of citing statistics that show they're more likely to be killed driving to events than participating in them. Even skydiving is less risky than driving America's highways.

Be certain, however, that he's playing it safe. If he's a bicyclist, for example, buy him a fancy helmet for his birthday and tell him how cool he looks in it. One recent study found that bicyclists who wear helmets are nearly 75 percent less likely to suffer head injuries than riders without helmets. Of the eleven fatalities in the study group, only one was helmeted. There's no excuse for anyone to climb on a bicycle without a helmet.

Unfortunately, men who do take up a sport often overdo it. Men over forty—particularly those who have been sedentary—should have a physical exam before taking up an athletic pursuit. Besides general health, the physician will be particularly interested in the condition of his heart and may suggest an exercise stress test, which measures the heart's reaction to exercise on a treadmill. It's the best way to get started in exercise without risking a heart attack.

If you are still anxious about his athletic endeavors, consider joining him. Not only will you fret less if you're there doing it with him, but he'll be particularly cautious if you're around. Some guys are overprotective, which can feel condescending even if they mean well. It may take some time to develop a healthy sporting relationship.

Many women believe that men eventually grow out of a love of physical risk-taking. Don't count on it. Sure, some high school football players become as placid as pandas by the time they're thirty. More men, however, level off for a while and then crescendo as they push toward that crisis time of middle age. Don't be surprised if your previously sensible forty-something fellow takes up rock climbing or joins a hockey league. If he selects his midlife crisis sport with care, he'll probably be a healthier, fitter, happier guy in the long run.

11

"You Look a Little Tense, Honey"

He's stressed, you're stressed, and it's getting worse. Nearly half the people interviewed in a 1994 study said that their stress levels had increased in the previous two years, and it sure feels as if the trend is continuing. And all this stress is making us sick.

Millions of years ago the human response to stress evolved to keep us alive. Our ancestors led lives punctuated occasionally by life-threatening crises. Over time, the human body developed an effective mechanism for surviving these sudden dangers; in a crisis, adrenaline and other hormones rush through the bloodstream to ready us for action. The chemicals push the heart rate up, constrict blood vessels, make blood more prone to clot, shut off blood flow to the digestive tract, mobilize energy stores, cut insulin production, and suppress reproductive hormones. We are instantly ready for "fight or flight."

These physical responses can be lifesavers when we face real danger, but they're not good for us when they constantly kick in under modern life's barrage of psychological and social pressures. When blood vessels stay constricted for a long time, they become less elastic, and blood pressure stays elevated permanently. This increases the risk of heart disease and stroke. Blood clots can block arteries. A digestive system deprived of blood is more likely to develop ulcers, irritable bowel syndrome, and gas. High glucose availability and suppressed insulin production can lead straight to diabetes. Low testosterone levels in a man have obvious consequences.

That set of symptoms and problems describes many of my patients. For example, Jack came to me because his libido was lagging, but during the initial interview I learned that he suffered from indigestion and lack of energy as well. Furthermore, his routine blood pressure test showed an elevated reading.

Jack was hoping for a dose of testosterone to get him going again, but instead we talked a little about his life—which turned out to be about 99 percent work. I suggested that he take a vacation—a real one!—and check back with me at the end of it. He objected that he was too busy to take a vacation. "Okay," I said, "consider it doctor's orders."

Most men don't understand that the effects of stress are cumulative and serious. Over time, an elevated level of the chemical cortisol increases the risk of diabetes, depression, cancer, heart attacks, stroke, high blood pressure, and low immunity. More than half of heart attack victims report they experienced an "extremely meaningful" psychological event in the twenty-four hours before their attack. Stress even increases cholesterol levels.

Naturally you don't want your man to suffer from these health problems. Consider also the effects of his stress on you. When his stress affects your relationship, the conflicts are likely to be harder on you than on him. A fascinating study has measured the chemicals released in men and women during and after a common type of altercation in which she wants a change and he simply refuses to engage. Often in relationship problems, the woman will see what's wrong, confront him about it, and demand remedial action. In response, he withdraws. I see this pattern in my office almost every day. A couple comes to see me, usually at her insistence, to get help with sexual problems. She has a lot to say, but he sits in stony silence. The study found that in situations like these, the man's portfolio of stress chemicals stays essentially unchanged, but the woman's levels of several stress chemicals, especially cortisol, jump up and may stay there for extended periods. You were pretty sure you felt worse than he did after an argument, and you were right. What's bothering him could make you sick.

I wish I could give directions to a Shangri-La where you and your guy could go to escape this stressful world, but the truth is there is stress in your future. I can tell you, though, how to manage the stress better.

Stress on the Job

When men are questioned in their calmer moments about the stress in their lives, it's clear that most of it stems from work—either their jobs or their fears about unemployment, changing jobs, or money. Only about a quarter say their stress comes from their family or a relationship.

Yet to admit that work is causing stress is not the American way. In most companies it's considered weak to succumb to the stresses of a job. Tough guys handle it and rise to the top. Since his employer probably won't help him with stress, you can make a big difference by helping him recognize the sources of stress in his job, then reduce or cope with them.

The number one way to manage workday stress is exercise, particularly aerobic exercise. Not only does working out take his mind off job pressures but after twenty to thirty minutes of aerobic exercise, he'll get a "runner's high," a feeling of tranquility caused by a release of chemicals called endorphins and lasting long after he finishes his workout. Believe me, the improvement can be profound. I like to run at 6:00 A.M. so I can get to the office early, relaxed and energized, while others are still fumbling for their coffee. It helps me stay a step ahead all day.

Exercise is hard to fit around many men's workdays, so I suggest that he make it fit *into* his workday. Walking with coworkers at lunchtime is one easy option, and taking the stairs instead of the elevator will make a difference. But I think his employer ought to be encouraging him to exercise—and even subsidizing it. Numerous studies have shown that an employer who spends $1.00 encouraging workers to exercise and avail themselves of preventive medicine saves at least $3.00 in health care costs and absenteeism.

One man I know is such a zealot about exercise that he's managed to persuade most of his immediate coworkers to follow suit. Of the ten people in his work group, six have joined his health club and two others are bicycling and swimming on their own. He tells me that since converting his coworkers to the wonders of exercise, workaday tensions have practically been eliminated, they've managed to meet all deadlines with relative ease, and they finished the most recent fiscal year under budget.

Besides exercising, your man also needs to find ways to reduce the types of stress that trigger the biggest release of hormones. Robert Sapolsky, a physiologist and stress researcher, explains in his wonderful book *Why Zebras Don't Get Ulcers* that unpredictable stress is particularly damaging. When we know it's coming but don't know when, we stay in a permanently stressed condition waiting for the other shoe to drop. Your partner may not be able to make all the stress on his job predictable, but communicating his plans and progress to superiors and coworkers may encourage them to inform him of theirs.

Stress stemming from lack of control is also destructive. It's important that he search for ways to increase his sense of control over his work. By simply asking him to tell you what he's doing and going to be doing at work, you'll be helping him organize his thoughts. Then suggest he pass along those great ideas to others. Be positive; focus on solutions rather than on problems.

Stress Busters

If he's talking about his day and complains about a particular source of stress, you can share one of these simple stress management techniques.

• **Close the door.** If noisy colleagues are getting on his nerves, suggest that he set aside at least an hour a day when he closes the door and concentrates. No door? Buy him a Walkman and headphones.

• **Take a break.** Backache and eyestrain worsen stress. It helps for him to stop at least once an hour, stand up, look out a window at distant objects, and touch his toes. Breaks increase productivity by 15 percent, so he needn't feel guilty.

• **Control the phone.** Constant interruptions when he's trying to focus on work can cause monumental stress. Sometimes it's okay to let his voice mail screen the calls. When he calls back, he'll have the control.

• **Make a list before leaving work.** If he writes down what needs to be accomplished the next day before going home, he can leave the work at work.

• **Breathe.** Under stress, breathing becomes shallow. Deep, slow breathing turns off the stress chemicals. Inhale, pause, and exhale to a count of four.

• **Call you.** Encourage him to give you a ring when the pressure mounts at the office. Just being there so he can vent will do wonders.

Social support on the job helps most men tolerate petty and not so petty injustices. The Dilbert comic strip phenomenon—the ability to laugh with colleagues about the sometimes absurd demands of the job—is the preferred coping technique of nearly three-quarters of all workers. Although seeing coworkers socially can be a risky proposition—particularly for people who work together closely—an occasional lunch away from the workplace can help your guy connect with his coworkers in ways that can help carry him through the annoyances of the workday. A beer after work with the guys isn't exactly a behavior you'd like to encourage, but as an occasional thing it may offer you great returns.

Sometimes the only way to protect one's well-being is quitting the job. When should a job be abandoned? A job that lacks predictability, control, and social support may deserve the take-it-and-shove-it approach. Stress on the job is nothing to be taken lightly. A study in Sweden found that lack of control on the job increased the risk of death from heart disease by 1.8 times, and lack of support on the job increased it 2.6 times. If at all possible, support him if he really needs to walk away.

Learning to Leave Work at Work

His job may create most of his stress, but the best opportunities for doing something about it occur away from work. There are as many strategies as there are individuals—stress and stress management are very personal things—but they all come down to finding activities that help him leave work at work. I'd like to introduce you to some techniques that have worked for others:

• **Take up a hobby.** An avocation is the perfect balance to a vocation. Perhaps he needs to indulge that urge to take up woodworking. Most stress-relieving hobbies involve doing something (often something repetitive) with the hands; there's truth in the old expression "Busy hands are happy hands." Competitive sports offer distraction and a chance to exercise. Gardening takes the mind off workaday worries while providing both exercise and healthy foods for the dinner table. Music has charms to soothe a savage beast.

• **Get a pet.** Pets distract us from our worries. Also, people with dogs walk more than those who don't have them. Petting an animal relieves stress in both owner and pet. Happy pet owners live longer after heart attacks and have lower blood pressure. Interestingly, one study of professionals who care for Alzheimer's disease patients found that men, but not women, who owned dogs were happier and less stressed than those who didn't have pets.

• **Have faith.** Religious beliefs can lower your stress when things go wrong in your life. For example, careful research has shown that parents of children with cancer do better if they can say to themselves, "This is a test from God. He chose us because He knew we could handle it." Also, support from fellow churchgoers makes a major difference for many people. Of course, faith doesn't have to come solely in the Judeo-Christian form. Meditative faiths such as Buddhism are equally able to reduce the effects of stress.

• **Play with him.** Many a workaholic has completely forgotten how to play. Somewhere deep inside there's still a child, and you can help find him. Can you talk your man into going dancing? It's great exercise and a wonderful stress reliever. No? Well, how about bowling, ice skating, or a round of miniature golf? Doing something just for fun puts work in its place.

- **Suggest a vacation.** One of the myths of American life is that a week or two of vacation will compensate for fifty or fifty-one weeks at a high-stress job. That's too much to ask of a vacation. But for a man who can't separate his life from his work, a vacation may be the only way to initiate the break. After a couple of weeks away, the rest of these techniques have a better chance of working. Of course, if he takes his cell phone and laptop to the beach every day, he's not really on vacation. Then there's the type who brags that he hasn't taken a vacation in years or thinks dire things will happen if he's gone more than a few days. Talk to him about the kind of vacation he'd find most relaxing, make your own wish list, and then plan a true vacation that you'll both love. Most important, do be sure you really get away. I have a friend who likes to go sailing in the Caribbean. Recently he said to me, "Don't tell anyone that I could have a cell phone with me. I tell them that they'll have to hail me by radio through a marine operator if they need me, and it'll take a few hours."
- **Try couple massage.** Unlike many cultures where communication includes touching, Americans are strictly hands off. Too bad, because human beings need touch. A relaxing, sensual way to put touching back in your lives is with massage. You don't have to be a masseuse or even have strong hands to give a great massage. If you want to learn some techniques, take a community education class together or read a book.
- **Encourage him to volunteer.** Something as simple as going along with you once a month to provide a meal at a homeless shelter will do wonders for his perspective on life. We need to care for others as much as we need to be cared for.
- **Look for support groups.** Whatever his particular problem, there's a support group out there to back him up. The benefits are real; cancer patients who join support groups live longer than those who go it on their own.
- **Meditate.** Meditation is a relaxation technique, not a religion. Through a class, audiotape, or book, he can learn this wonderful way to relax completely.

Professional Help with Stress

You can help him improve his ability to manage stress, but if stress is making him anxious, angry, or depressed, he may need professional counseling. He can also learn techniques from a therapist such as autogenics and biofeedback, as well as other strategies for coping with stress.

While you are working on his stress, watch your own levels carefully. You'll do neither of you any good if you stress yourself out working on his stress.

Stretch Out the Stress

Tension builds up in unexpected areas in the body, so it's best for him to perform this entire routine from top to bottom. Still, even one stretch is better than none.

1. **Face and scalp.** Raise your eyebrows, then open your eyes as wide as possible. Follow with an openmouthed yawn. Repeat several times.

2. **Neck.** Roll your head toward your right or left shoulder without raising the shoulder. Hold for ten seconds, then roll the head slowly forward and around to the other shoulder. Hold for ten seconds, then roll back. (Don't roll the head backward!)

3. **Shoulders.** Lift one arm over your head, then bend it over your shoulder and reach down your back. Put your other arm behind your back and reach up to try to make your fingers meet. Switch sides and repeat.

4. **Upper back.** Standing with your feet shoulder-width apart, grasp both your elbows in front and raise them as high as your forehead. Slowly bend forward, stretching your arms and neck outward. Hold at the lowest possible position for ten seconds.

5. **Lower back.** Either sitting in a chair or lying faceup on the floor, raise your knees one at a time to your chest and hold for ten seconds.

6. **Backs of thighs.** Find a desk, table, or counter about hip height. Raise one leg and place its heel on the surface. Bend your torso toward the foot and hold for ten seconds. Repeat for the other leg.

7. **Fronts of thighs.** Holding on to a table or counter with your right hand, bend your left leg. Use your free hand to grasp your ankle and pull your foot up gently behind you. Hold for ten seconds and repeat on the other side.

8. **Calves.** Standing three or four feet from a wall, place the palms of both hands against it. Bend one knee and step forward so that the back of the other leg stretches. Hold for ten seconds without bouncing. Repeat.

12

More Than the Blues, More Than a Temper

We all have emotional ups and downs. At times we may temporarily despair over one of life's setbacks, and at other times we may bristle in anger at an injustice we've suffered. Anyone who stays totally on an even keel day in and day out either leads a charmed life or isn't tuned in to reality.

Some people, however, don't bounce back easily from life's injustices. Because of a combination of genetic heritage, life experiences, and, as we're increasingly learning, biochemical imbalances, what some of us can shrug off dominates the lives of others. Seemingly minor problems can trigger deep depression or explosive anger.

Men are much more likely than women to express their extreme emotions violently. Each year nearly 25,000 men—four times as many as women—take their own lives, and it has been estimated that as many as 5 million men each year hit their partners. These are truly alarming numbers.

Paul Kivel of the Oakland Men's Project believes that men's violence stems from the need to be in control, which he feels is the most fundamental lesson American culture teaches boys. From an early age boys are taught to control their bodies by being tough and ignoring pain; to control their emotions by hiding them, even from themselves; and to control others in order to succeed.

Of course, the very notion that anyone can be totally in control is absurd. In the workplace there's always someone higher up the totem pole. We can campaign, lobby, and vote, but we still won't control our communities. We can win an occasional victory on the tennis court, but there's always a better player around. Most of us manage to work with and accept our lack of complete control, but some men don't handle it well. The "control freak" may consider his family a last chance to exert control—if not over you, then over the children or at least the dog. He may attempt it by authoritarianism, by emotional coercion, by financial extortion, or, if he becomes truly desperate, by violence.

Other men with control problems direct their anger toward themselves. They become anxious or depressed, start drinking heavily or abusing drugs, and may contemplate suicide. Often a man will vacillate between internally and externally directed violence in a cycle of abusing himself, alcohol, and his partner. Depression and domestic violence may well be two sides of the same problem: men feeling they are losing control.

If your man is depressive or abusive, you didn't make him that way. You may feel that you're the focus of his problem, but you're just the scapegoat. He has a medical problem. It can be treated, and he can get better. But your wanting it isn't enough; he has to want to get better, too. You can help to some extent, but he has to accept responsibility for his problems. And you must look out for yourself.

When the Blues Turn Black

More than 6 million Americans suffer from episodes of depression each year. In any six-month period, 3.5 percent of American men have at least one period of depression.

Medically, clinical depression is defined as a period of at least two weeks in which a person shows at least one of the first two signs and five signs altogether in the following list:

- **Depressed mood**
- **Loss of interest or pleasure in usual activities**
- Feelings of worthlessness or excessive or inappropriate guilt
- Inability to concentrate or make decisions
- Fatigue or loss of energy
- Appetite change or weight loss
- Sleeping too little or too much
- Jerky or slow physical reactions
- Unusual and persistent pains, such as headache
- Recurrent thoughts of death or suicide

Because the effects of depression vary so much, the condition often goes unnoticed. About 80 percent of depressed people could be successfully treated, but only about 30 percent seek help. Suicide is too often the result. More than 60 percent of people who take their own lives each year are clinically depressed.

When the Symptoms Don't Quite Fit

Clinical, also called "major," depression is just one of the categories of depressive illness. Two other types of depression, with different symptoms, may affect your loved one.

Dysthmia produces less pronounced symptoms than major depression but may last for years, until a person actually forgets what it's like to feel good. Dysthmia can also be mixed with periods of major depression.

Bipolar disorder, or manic-depressive illness, causes cycles between depression and elation. During the depressive period, the person shows the signs of depression. During the manic phase, the person may experience insomnia, excessive energy, overconfidence, racing thoughts, or wild behavior. The switch from mania to depression may take place slowly or quickly, and the extremes may be separated by normal periods. Bipolar disease is recognized even less often than clinical depression; only about a quarter of people with the problem receive treatment.

Men are especially unlikely to receive adequate treatment for depression. In his revealing book *I Don't Want to Talk About It*, Terrence Real discusses what he calls *covert depression*—a largely male condition. The psychotherapist believes that depression is not diagnosed because men are rewarded in our society for withholding emotional expression. He cites studies showing overdiagnosis of depression in women and underdiagnosis in men because men won't express their unhappiness and because therapists expect women to be depressed. Real argues convincingly that men get depressed in different ways from women—ways that may go unnoticed or, at least, are not seen as depression. In men, numbness and detachment—or their polar opposite, violence—are more likely than tears or emotional outbursts.

Frankly, depression isn't easy to identify in anyone. First of all, depressed people of either sex only rarely recognize their situation as a medical problem and seek professional help; men make it worse by seeing the very act of asking for help as an admission of weakness. Armed with the list of symptoms, you're much more likely to recognize his depression than he is. Still, he probably won't make it easy to notice them. In a society where, as Paul Simon put it, "I'd rather be a hammer than a nail," expressing anguish isn't a male characteristic.

Be especially watchful for symptoms if one or both of his parents had depression. If one parent has been depressed, the odds are one in four that the children will develop depression by age seventeen, if both parents were depressed, the odds rise to even.

If your partner or anyone else you're close to is exhibiting signs of depression—and especially if he's talking about suicide—don't assume that he's merely looking for sympathy or that it will pass. Call his doctor right away. Early and effective treatment appears to reduce the likelihood of recurrence of depression. Left untreated, depression often accelerates from a temporary reaction to major stresses to a more or less permanent reaction to even minor stresses.

Illness and Depression

A large number of people with physical problems suffer from depression. About 20 percent of those who have heart attacks subsequently become depressed, making them significantly less likely to recover from their physical problem. Likewise, 25 to 30 percent of Parkinson's disease patients develop depression, and the number rises as high as 35 percent among stroke victims. If someone you love has a major health problem, be on the lookout for signs of depression.

Treatment options for depression have expanded greatly in the past decade. The most famous of the new drugs, Prozac, has been both hailed as a wonder drug and derided as pop psychology for yuppies. The fact is, it's neither. Prozac is just one of a variety of antidepressant medications, none of which has been shown to be more effective than the others. Its popularity among doctors stems more from its lack of side effects in most people than from superior performance. (Sleep disturbances, lowered libido, and difficulty achieving orgasm are the most common side effects in men.) Prozac belongs to a class of medicines called selective seratonin reuptake inhibitors (SSRIs). Other older, equally effective classifications include tricyclic antidepressants (TCAs) and monoamine oxidase (MAO) inhibitors.

The key to proper pharmaceutical treatment of depression is to find an antidepressant that works well at a dosage which produces minimal side effects. It's important to know that antidepressant medicines take at least two weeks to become effective and that it often takes some experimentation to find the right drug at the right dose. So during the early weeks the depressed person needs to be watched closely by both physician and loved ones for signs of problems. And remember, pills don't guarantee success. Medical science still understands little about what makes antidepressant medicines work—and for 15 to 20 percent of people, they don't.

Although "talk therapy" for depression isn't emphasized as much as it once was, it is still vitally important for a depressed person. And it's nearly as effective. About 70 percent of people recover from their depression with psychotherapy, versus 80 percent with medications. More important, psychotherapy may help people for whom drugs don't work well, and eventually it may allow medication to be discontinued. Whether therapy takes the form of individual counseling, group therapy, or psychoanalysis, it can reduce his sense of isolation, help him recognize and manage sources of stress, and simply provide nonjudgmental support. Encourage your depressed partner to seek counseling; it's likely to improve the odds and speed of his recovery.

Living with a depressed person can be very stressful even if you recognize that you didn't cause the problem. You'll probably feel helpless because there seems to be so little you can do to improve his mood. Once he's admitted that he's depressed and needs help, what role can you play in his recovery?

Most counselors will ask that you be present for at least some of the therapy sessions. Your participation can not only help him recover more quickly and thoroughly but can also help protect you from being drawn into his web of depression. You'll learn how to maintain as normal a relationship as possible during his treatment—all the while acknowledging that he is suffering. During this time it will be especially important to remind him of the affection and respect you hold for him—feelings we all too often fail to express. Negatives may best be put on the back burner for the time being. You can also encourage him to be more physically active. Exercise is often an integral part of the prescription for treating depression. Finally, don't expect him to just snap out of it. Depression can be beat, but it takes time.

The Abusive Relationship

When a man experiences powerlessness in the outside world, he may resort to a variety of means to control his family. He may use physical violence or emotional abuse. He may exert his power over you with intimidation, emotional manipulation, sex, money, threats, isolation, rejection, or even the children. Every example of physical abuse also involves emotional abuse, and the frequency of emotional abuse alone is a great unknown. Spouse abuse is more than black eyes and broken bones.

In their book *Before It's Too Late*, Robert Ackerman and Susan Pickering list a series of questions to ask yourself if you suspect you're involved in an abusive relationship:

• Has he hit you or hurt you physically?
• Does he sometimes drink too much and become physically or emotionally abusive?
• Does he threaten you?
• Does he blame you for problems in your relationship?
• Does he call you a nag for wanting to discuss problems in your relationship?
• Does he accuse you of flirting?
• Does he suspect you've become involved with other people?
• Does he ever follow you or check on your whereabouts?
• Is he often late without letting you know he will be?
• Does he forbid or discourage your outside activities?
• Does he embarrass you in front of others?
• Does he get angry if you disagree with him?
• Does he criticize your looks or apparel?
• Does he insist on always driving the car?
• Does he clam up or withhold affection when he doesn't win?
• Does he tell you he "needs his freedom"?
• Does he control the money—forbidding you to have your own checking account or giving you an allowance?
• Does he use sex to quell your doubts about the relationship?
• Is he uninterested in what happened in your day?
• Does he reward you with presents for "being good"?
• Does he use a derogatory nickname for you?
• Does he expect you to be home when he gets home?
• Is he angry or uncomfortable when you get positive attention?
• Does he disregard or demean your accomplishments?
• Does he minimize or make fun of your feelings?
• Do you often feel that he's too critical of you?
• Does he flirt in front of you?
• Does he try to make you feel sorry for him?
• Does he find fault with your friends or other family?

Answering yes to more than five of these questions suggests that control plays a role in your relationship; the more yes answers you gave, the more likely you're suffering abusive control from your partner. At the lower end of the scale, counseling may be in order to get your relationship back on track. As the tally of abuse mounts—and anytime physical abuse is involved—you and he need help right away.

To be quite frank, therapists tell me that if a man is physically abusive, his spouse will probably have to leave, even if only temporarily. As long as she's in the house, the cycle of control will probably not stop. Leaving is no easy step. The woman must face fears of retribution and of her unknown future. However bad the situation is at home, at least it's no surprise. And often there's still a good deal of love around—interspersed with pain. She may hope that he'll spontaneously get better (which rarely happens). Other hurdles to leap include finances, the loss of physical and emotional connection, the effect on the children, separation from friends, embarrassment, and potentially the abrogation of marriage vows. None of these challenges is easy, and together they're more than many women can face.

Fortunately, there is support. First, she can get a court order called Protection from Abuse (PFA), which forbids him from harassing her. Unfortunately, abusive men are rarely jailed for more than twenty-four hours, so the effectiveness of a PFA depends largely on how supportive the local police force can or will be. A local Legal Aid office can help a woman get a PFA and inform her of her other rights. Women's shelters offer both protection and support. For women without friends or family to back them up, shelters are an excellent resource. It takes support to make the jump, but it's vital that a battered woman protect herself by getting out.

If recovery is possible, it has to begin with the man becoming willing to seek help. Family, friends, and clergy may help bring him to this stage. More likely, though, according to Terrence Real, he will get help simply because he wants you back. He knows he has to do something, though he may not know yet what that something is.

Next comes the stage of owning his behavior—admitting that he's the source of the problem, not you, and that he needs help to get over it. This is progress, but he still has a long way to go. If drinking is involved, that problem has to be addressed as well.

If he succeeds in changing, he'll probably be breaking a chain that has continued in his family for generations. Many abusers were themselves victims of abuse in their past. I like to think that we men are making progress in understanding that masculinity isn't something we earn by victimizing others, but the numbers of abused women tell me that more work must be done. Men lack the assurance in their masculinity that women seem to find in their femininity; I think it is because we devote so much effort to denying an important part of ourselves.

To me, one of the most powerful arguments for embracing our more emotional, compassionate, caring side is to benefit our sons. There's little that is more important than breaking the vicious cycle of abusive behavior both toward women and toward our fellow men. As Terrence Real put it, "Boys don't hunger for fathers who will model traditional mores of masculinity. They hunger for fathers who will rescue them from it."

Part III

"Can't Help Lovin' That Man of Mine"

13

Men Unzipped

Three engineers were arguing about the nature of God. The first said that God is a mechanical engineer—look at the intricate joints and bones and how they move. The second argued that God is an electrical engineer—look at the incredible brain and nervous system. But the third engineer said no, God *has* to be a civil engineer—who else would run a waste-disposal pipeline through a great recreational area?

Indeed. Yet the male urogenital system is a marvel. To most women *and* men, it's also a mystery. It's obvious that a penis can become erect, but how? When it doesn't, why not? Where does semen come from? And what is a prostate, anyway? Many men have questions and concerns about penis size, masturbation, circumcision, even nighttime erections. It's fascinating and enlightening to learn how it all works.

From the Kidneys on Down

Let's take a tour. We'll start with the urinary system, just above the place where the male and female systems start to differ. (When I take men on this tour, I usually start with the focus of their attention and work backward. If you are a tour guide for your man, you may want to go "upstream.")

Like you, a man has two kidneys that, among other things, filter impurities from blood and produce urine to carry away waste products. From the kidneys the urine travels through the ureters to the bladder, where it's stored until he urinates. Here's where the differences begin.

Urine passes from the bladder to the outside of the body through the urethra. In a woman, this tube is only one to two inches long, but in a man, it's four to six inches long, running the length of his penis. In a man, a muscle called the bladder neck holds the bladder closed so that urine doesn't move into the urethra until he wants it to. Just below the bladder neck, the urethra is surrounded by the prostate gland. In a thirty-year-old guy, the prostate is usually the size of a walnut, but with age it often enlarges. An enlarged prostate may squeeze the urethra, reducing or even eliminating urine flow.

We know some of the things the prostate does, but we're far from knowing all its purposes. (A man with a problem prostate will tell you it's of no use at all.) The prostate consists of both glandular and muscular tissue. The glandular tissues secrete prostatic fluid, which makes up one-quarter to one-third of the volume of semen. The muscle tissues, by bearing down on the urethra, can prevent semen from flowing upstream toward the bladder or urine from flowing downward. (Tension in this muscle at the wrong times can produce the same sorts of problems as an enlarged prostate.) Whatever else the prostate may do, a guy can get along just fine without one. The most significant effect of removal is that during ejaculation, part of the semen can go back into the bladder (retrograde ejaculation) since the muscular tissue is no longer there to control flow. (As we'll discuss in chapter 20, there are also other potential side effects of prostate surgery.)

After passing the prostate, the urethra goes through the diaphragm that separates the bladder and prostate from the external genitalia. Then it runs through the penis. The urine exits at the meatus.

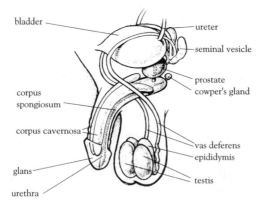

The Reproductive System

This portion of the journey, which is a bit more fun, begins in the testes. There is a common misconception that the testes provide the fluid that makes up semen. In fact, although the testes do produce all the *sperm* in semen, sperm account for less than 5 percent of the overall volume. The testes also produce between 60 and 65 percent of testosterone, the male sex hormone, and secrete it into the bloodstream. (The rest is produced in the adrenal gland.) Testosterone gives men (and women) their sex drive, makes erections possible, controls male characteristics such as facial hair, and serves other purposes, too.

Testes begin life well up inside the abdomen and gradually descend as the fetus nears birth. In rare cases the testes fail to descend outside the abdominal cavity before birth. Undescended testes need to be surgically corrected. Otherwise, they will fail to produce sperm and will greatly increase the risk of testicular cancer.

The testes are inside the scrotum (one layer of skin and six of muscle). The scrotum and the cremasteric muscle (attached from the abdomen to each testicle) can raise and lower the testes to maintain the ideal temperature for sperm production (two degrees cooler than the body). The cremasteric muscle may also raise the testes in response to fright—a protective response—or during arousal. (Interestingly, this doesn't seem to happen to animals.) In some men the testes actually disappear inside the abdomen. This isn't dangerous as long as it's temporary.

Although more men worry about penis size than testicle size, it's not unusual for a man to be concerned that small testes mean he's less manly. Pass it along from someone who's seen plenty: Testes come in a wide variety of sizes, and bigger does not mean more virile. Also, one is usually larger than the other, and one will usually hang lower in the scrotum.

Sperm start off in the testes in tiny tubular cells that produce spermatocytes (just as a woman's ovaries produce oocytes). They mature there for more than seventy days. When they emerge, they're still not ready for prime time. They need to grow stronger in the epididymis, an assemblage of tubes attached to the back of each testicle. Completely uncoiled, an epididymis would be twenty feet long, but it is compacted into a half-inch-wide and an inch long. Sperm production varies depending on the frequency of ejaculation. A man who is sexually inactive produces fewer. The number actually ejaculated varies quite a bit, but an average number might be around 60 million.

Once they reach the end of the epididymis, sperm are mature and able to swim actively (called motility) by wiggling their tails. They then travel up the vas deferens, tubes that are one to two feet long and about the thickness of large spaghetti. The vas are the pipelines that are cut and blocked off during vasectomy. The vas deferens and surrounding blood vessels form the spermatic cord.

Just before reaching the prostate gland, the vas deferens widen into the ampulla, where sperm wait for the opportunity to be ejaculated. The seminal vesicles, which are behind the prostate and bladder, supply a fructose (sugar) mixture to the ejaculatory fluid to support the sperm on their reproductive journey. Thus the fluid called semen consists of sperm from the testes, prostatic fluid from prostatic ducts, and seminal fluid from the seminal vesicles.

Before the semen spurts from the urethra, the Cowper's gland secretes a small amount of watery fluid into the urethra. This is usually present at the tip of the penis during arousal and prior to ejaculation. Although we're not certain what purpose it serves, the Cowper's gland secretions probably lubricate the inside of the urethra to make way for the semen.

Shortly before ejaculation, semen cues up in the urethra. In the pelvic area, increasing muscle tension creates a feeling that ejaculation is imminent and irreversible. Signals from a nerve center in the spinal column go out to muscles in the pelvic area. The bladder neck closes to prevent the semen from going into the bladder. Then the muscles that surround the portion of the penis inside the abdomen contract powerfully to expel the semen.

Shortly after ejaculation, the components of the semen change so they can protect the sperm in the woman's vagina. If one sperm finds an egg moving through the fallopian tube, the result is parenthood.

Erection

You may have noticed that something was missing from the discussion of ejaculation—an erect penis. That's because ejaculation and erection are completely distinct functions. They are controlled by nerve centers in different parts of the spine, under direction of the brain, and one can happen without the other. Yes, he can ejaculate without having an erection. Erections are useful, though, so let's look at how they work.

Underneath the skin of the penis an elastic layer called the tunica albuginea encloses three cylinders, two composed entirely of blood vessel tissue and one on the inside through which urine and semen pass. All three of these cylinders extend inside the abdomen—about one-third of the penis is actually inside the body—and are surrounded by muscles. Arteries, vessels that bring blood rich in nutrients and oxygen from the heart, run up the center of the two outer cylinders. Branches in the arteries feed blood to storage areas in the cylinders called lacunae (lakes). Veins, the vessels that carry used blood back to the heart, exit the lakes, pass through the tunica, and run back inside the abdomen under the skin.

Getting an erection is like filling up a tire at the service station except that the penis fills with blood rather than air. To get the job done, a man needs a good control switch (brain), well-insulated wires (nerves), a strong compressor (the heart), an adequate supply line (arteries), and a tire without leaks (the penis). If any of these components is defective, he has a flat tire.

As a man goes about his normal daily activities, the supply lines (arteries) are relatively small, and very little blood enters the lakes. Why? Here's the tricky part. Blood flow remains minimal, just enough to keep tissues alive, because muscle tissue in the penis stays tense. I know it sounds odd, but a flaccid penis requires tense muscles, although he's never aware of those muscles. Within the walls of the arteries and lakes they prevent the lakes from filling with blood. The blood that does enter the penis to nourish tissues flows through without meeting much resistance.

For twenty-one or twenty-two hours of the average man's day, the muscles stay tense and his penis stays neatly tucked away. Three things can flip the switch. One, some sexual thought—of you, of course—might enter his mind, causing nerve impulses to travel down his spinal column. Two, direct stimulation of his penis can cause nerve impulses to travel a different pathway up to the brain and then back down to the spine. Three, when he is sound asleep, his brain may trigger the impulses that bring on erection. Most men have two to four erections lasting fifteen to thirty minutes every night while they sleep. Many men think that they become erect during the night because they need to urinate (the so-called pee hard-on), but actually they're having a normal nocturnal erection. I've never met a man who told me he gets erections during the day when he needs to urinate. This nighttime activity brings oxygen to the tissues of the penis, helping to keep things working correctly.

Whatever the instigator, when the call goes out for an erection, a complex neurochemical process begins. Nerve impulses from the spinal column, mediated by the brain, cause nerve endings in the penis to release chemicals, including nitric oxide. Nitric oxide stimulates an enzyme called guanylate cyclase, which, in turn, promotes the accumulation of cyclic guanosine monophosphate (cGMP) inside the smooth muscle cells in the penis. cGMP forces calcium out of the muscle cells, leading to relaxation. The lower the calcium concentration, the greater the relaxation. Thus, the arteries can expand, increasing blood flow; the muscle cells and supportive tissues of the lakes fill with blood, and an erection is on its way. (A second set of nerves can release chemicals that cause those muscles to tense up again, quickly dispatching an erection. As you'll learn in a later chapter, when this switch gets flipped at the wrong time, it's a problem.)

As the lakes expand, they compress the veins that normally carry blood out of the penis, dramatically reducing the outward flow. Pressures inside the penis exceed the peak pumping pressure of the heart, then go even higher near the peak of arousal when the muscles that surround the body contract. Squeezing the head of the penis—primarily with the vagina—may further increase blood pressure. In any event, as long as the switch stays on, the pressure stays high enough, and leaks do not develop, his penis will stay inflated.

Hormones Make the Man

That's *how* erections work, but it's also worth considering *why*. Although they don't directly cause an erection, hormones secreted by the testes and adrenal gland control our interest in sex and our level of arousal. We don't know whether these hormones work on the brain, the genitals, or both, but they clearly are indispensable to a vibrant sex life.

The most important hormone for men is testosterone. It controls secondary sexual characteristics, bone density, and sexual desire. (Testosterone levels also control a woman's level of interest in sex, but because the hormone plays so many other roles in a man, he has ten to fifteen times more.) Despite testosterone's importance, lower levels usually aren't the cause of sexual problems. Even later in life when men produce less testosterone, 80 percent still have levels in the normal range. (We'll talk more about this in chapter 19, "Mastering Midlife"). However, sexual desire, erections, and ejaculation are controlled by a cocktail of chemicals, and excess or lack of any one can interfere with what comes naturally.

The level of testosterone seldom stays steady in men or women, so sex drive varies. A man's testosterone level peaks at about eight in the morning and hits its low point about ten at night. Although there's quite a bit of variation from guy to guy, on average the peak is about 50 percent higher than the valley. Testosterone levels also vary with the seasons. They're highest in the early fall. Perhaps this pattern evolved because late spring used to be the best time to bear children. As already noted, a man's testosterone levels decline with age, beginning in his late forties.

Circumcision

The practice of removing the foreskin from the penis of a newborn male goes back to ancient times. Jewish and Muslim groups turned circumcision into a ritual more than four thousand years ago. Today at least half of all newborn males in the United States (1.25 million boys each year) are circumcised within a few days of birth. In Canada and Australia the number is between 30 and 40 percent. Circumcision is relatively rare in England, Scandinavia, and Japan. The wide variation in acceptance says a lot about the efficacy of the practice, and it also hints that circumcision can be a highly emotional issue for some men. To the father of a newborn the most important factor may be a desire to have his son "look like me" or "look like the other boys."

Medically, circumcision has merits. Uncircumcised males are ten to twenty times more likely to get urinary tract infections during the first few years of life, although the problem is rare anyway (only 2 percent of boys). Likewise, penile cancer occurs almost exclusively in the uncircumcised. Once again, the problem affects few males (1 in 100,000) and is probably linked to poor hygiene. (Penile cancer is rare in Japan and Scandinavia despite very low circumcision rates.) Uncircumcised men may also be more susceptible to sexually transmitted diseases and more likely to transmit them (or yeast infections) to their partners. Of course, problems of the foreskin, such as balanitis (inflammation) or phimosis (inability to retract during erection), happen only to the uncircumcised. On the minus side, like any surgery, circumcision carries a risk of infection and bleeding, and the procedure is painful.

Some men believe that circumcision may lead to premature ejaculation. There is no medical proof for this claim, and I have found no association in my practice. Nonetheless, some men believe fervently that circumcision has harmed them sexually. A grassroots group called RECAP even advocates stretching skin on the penis to mimic the lost foreskin.

It's not easy to make a decision about circumcision for your male children— unless, of course, a ritual is part of your religion. You and the child's father should make the choice together after talking with your pediatrician. An adult who wishes he were or weren't circumcised is another matter. Although circumcision of an adult man may be called for if he has a foreskin problem, he won't recover from the surgery as quickly as a newborn. Recovery will include some discomfort, about a week off work, and six weeks without intercourse. Unless there's a medical reason or an intense emotional one, I don't recommend it. Restoring foreskins is even more difficult. To my knowledge there is no practical way of doing it. Counseling is a better approach.

Is It Big Enough?

You can't imagine how much some guys worry that their penis isn't big enough. They stay anxious even after they are assured that size has little to do with satisfying a woman. It doesn't help them to learn that the average erect penis is a little over five inches long and that the average deviation is only a little more than an inch. It doesn't assuage their fears to learn that flaccid size doesn't predict erect size.

I've found that men with this obsession are less concerned about what a woman might think than about what other men will think. Men are often more worried about the locker room and group shower than the bedroom. The differences are magnified in their minds because the difference between flaccid and erect length varies a lot from man to man. Most men also think of an erection as an on or off proposition rather than a range of sizes. When I work with a man who has an erection problem, we rate his erections on a scale of one to ten. An erection of one is no response, five is sufficient for penetration, and ten is the most rigid erection he's ever had. A lightbulb often goes on when he begins to understand that it's a matter of degree.

Is a penis ever too small? Some doctors say it's too small anytime a man thinks it is. This attitude has had some unfortunate results. A California doctor performed about three thousand penile augmentations before being shut down by the California Medical Board. There are serious questions about both the effectiveness and safety of procedures to increase penis size. One critic has claimed that the complication rates approach 20 percent.

Three experts on the topic of penis length—Drs. Hunter Wessells, Tom Lue, and Jack McAninch of the University of California, San Francisco—have stated that augmentation should not even be considered for any man whose erect penis is longer than three inches, and they decline to perform surgical procedures on any man. They recommend that a man who wants a longer penis lose weight since the fat pad just above the penis in the abdomen swallows some of the length of the penis. The depth of that fat tends to increase with age until it hides more than an inch of the penis.

Needless to say, the size of his equipment may be a touchy subject. You'd do well to be cautious about bringing it up, and complimentary if it seems appropriate. Until the day my colleagues and I can talk men out of concentrating so much on the penis, size will remain a sensitive issue for quite a few men.

Solo Sex

Although for obvious reasons it's difficult to get reliable information about the practice of masturbation, most surveys have found that a large majority of men masturbate, perhaps over 90 percent, even if they have a satisfying sexual relationship with their partner. Chances are, therefore, that your man masturbates at least occasionally. If he does, it does not mean he's in any way displeased with you. Look at it this way: Even the most perfect couple won't always have parallel sexual desires. There may be times when you're interested and he isn't, and vice versa.

Ejaculation is healthful. It reduces stress and anxiety, and gets rid of fluids, which is good for the prostate. I often see men whose prostate problems stem from a change in ejaculatory patterns. What's more, sexual excitement helps keep tissues healthy (in both of you). New studies show that unused penises may shrink somewhat owing to muscular atrophy.

When you're unavailable, masturbation is certainly a better choice than the other outlets around town. Masturbation is only a problem if it takes the place of partner-based sex and begins to form a barrier to a loving relationship.

Durable but Not Unbreakable

I'm fond of telling men that they won't wear their penis out. Regular use is good maintenance. It is possible, however, to damage a penis. Bending an erect penis can cause immediate and serious damage or small injuries that can lead to later problems. Athletic sex ought to be practiced with caution. In particular, intercourse with the woman on top can cause a fracture if there's insufficient lubrication or the penis fails to go where it's supposed to. Penile fracture ruptures the outer wall of the chamber in the penis, and immediate surgery is necessary to preserve potency. Smaller injuries, ones that may not even be noticed at the time, may cause Peyronie's disease, bent penis (see chapter 15).

Considering the intricacies of sexuality, intercourse, fertility, and reproduction, it's a wonder how well it all works. Sex with a loving partner is nature's gift. Enjoy it to the fullest!

14

The Answers Aren't in
Playboy

W hat is it about men and sex that supports an entire wall of sleazy magazines at the newsstand? I think those R-rated and X-rated glossies sell because they make sex look simple. In the *Playboy* world, all the women are attractive and willing, and there's no relationship baggage. Sex doesn't have the daunting complications of emotion, commitment, or reproduction, let alone the risk of disease.

It's not fair to pick on the girlie magazines, though, as the Larry Flynts of the world have only refined and concentrated a view of sex that's also shown by television, movies, and advertising—because sex sells. Not real sex but *simple* sex in which all the men are muscular and handsome and have penises that go up like electric garage doors, and all the women are buxom, blond, and orgasmic.

Real sex is anything but simple. When it's good, it's a sharing of pleasures and emotions and commitment. Men who let their vision of simple sex rule their affairs chase good sex but never find it. They don't understand that good sex requires much more than a hard penis and a place to put it. In fact, there are many male myths that get in the way of good sex.

The Twelve Male Myths About Sex

In his book *New Male Sexuality*, my friend and colleague Dr. Bernie Zilbergeld identifies a dozen male myths about sex. Each is a barrier to good sexual relationships between men and women. You've probably seen most of these myths in action, but a few may surprise you. Here they are, with some advice I've added on how to help your man move beyond them.

Myth 1. Men are liberated about sex.

On the contrary, most American men feel quite uncomfortable talking openly about sex. This stems from men's fear that someone will find out they don't know it all. It's difficult to change when you think you're already there—and, furthermore, if you don't want to talk about it.

Myth 2. A real man doesn't express his feelings.

This fundamental male belief is the most harmful myth. As we discussed in chapter 2, men don't want to express emotions because they don't want to be vulnerable. Until a man learns to share his feelings, true sexual intimacy is impossible. The foundation of a good relationship and good sex is trust. It takes time to build trust. Trust him with your feelings, try to make him feel safe, then it's up to him.

Myth 3. All touching is sexual.

Men have a tough time telling sex from nonsex. Nonsexual touch is a fundamental human need. It soothes us and makes us feel cared for. Adults need to be held and touched just as much as small children do. One way to help your partner experience nonsexual touch is taking a couples massage class. Each of you will learn how to make the other feel good physically without being explicitly sexual. Even if he fails to see it as an end in itself, massage will offer both of you a prelude for sex, a time to become accustomed to touching and to relax. The more you become used to touching each other, the more the great divide between nonsexual and sexual will close.

Myth 4. A man is always interested in and ready for sex.

As silly as it may seem to you, a man can believe that he's substandard if he thinks everyone else but him is having sex 3.2 times a week. I'm sure you've experienced times when your partner's sexual advance seemed halfhearted. Did you worry that you weren't looking good to him? I hope you considered that he might still have been thinking about the hard day he had at work. Men won't admit that they're not up for sex because they're tired or distracted. They need to be less tough on themselves.

Myth 5. A real man performs in sex.

Too many men have sex to express not caring or even lust but their manliness. Obsessed with performance, they reduce sex to hardware and measurements and staying power. Ironically, when a man's "performance" declines with age, the couple's sexual satisfaction may well increase. He may not be able to have sex numerous times in one evening, but without the extreme urgency of youth, he may become more patient, thoughtful, and interested in the moment. Time can do a lot to cure a man of the performance obsession. You can help him get there sooner by telling him often that you're quite satisfied with him. A little positive feedback can ease his performance anxiety.

Myth 6. Sex is centered on a hard penis and what is done with it.
Many a man never gets over the fixation on the penis that's a universal part of being an adolescent male. To fully enjoy the sexual experience, a grown-up needs to stop ignoring the other 95 percent of his body, including the most important sex organ of all, his brain. A woman can also buy into this myth but with a different result. She may know that an erect penis isn't necessary or even ideally suited to her pleasure, but it becomes a sort of thermometer of his ardor. She thinks: no erection, no affection. In reality, erections can be cued by a number of psychological or physical stimuli. They need not have anything to do with love, though it's nice when they do.

Myth 7. Sex equals intercourse.
Good sex is more than just a meeting of the genitals. Men and women can share pleasure and closeness with their hands, eyes, ears, and minds, too. The more ways we share, the bigger the experience. Intercourse is important, but without the other delights, it's just a reproductive act. Many men tend to be goal-oriented about sex, and it's not easy to get them to slow down and enjoy the scenery. It will help him to know he's going to get there eventually. Planning time together, instead of fitting it in when other obligations allow, takes the pressure off. A scheduled candlelight dinner, perhaps followed by a warm bath, gives you both the opportunity to anticipate sex and the time to slow down and enjoy each other's company.

Myth 8. A man should always be able to give his partner an orgasm.
Women *have* orgasms; men don't *give* them orgasms. He may not see it that way. He may consider it his duty to make sure you have one. It's wonderful that he's concerned about your pleasure, but he needs to learn that an orgasm is not the only measure of success. Will it help to assure him that it doesn't really matter to you if you come every time? Not likely. He may only feel less important to you. Instead, he needs to feel successful in other, less directly sexual ways. What other ways can he help you feel good? Do you like to have your hair brushed? Ask. Is there a particular place on your back that itches

and is hard to reach? Let him scratch it for you. An orgasm is just one of the pleasures we can share.

Myth 9. Good sex requires that the man have an orgasm.
Men think sex and ejaculation are synonymous. Why? An automatic response of the nervous system is not good sex. For a man, particularly when he's young or middle-aged, *lack* of ejaculation is unlikely to be a concern. As a man grows older, though, ejaculation may not always be inevitable, and aside from reproduction, there's no reason that it should be. Once again, fixation on goals can get in the way of enjoying the process. As they grow older, many men are surprised (and delighted) to learn that sex isn't a one-act play that unfolds the same way each time. They discover that there is a variety of sexual responses, and that adds to their experience. The sooner a man can get there, the more he and his partner will benefit.

Myth 10. Men don't have to listen to women during sex.
He needs to consider that you mean what you say. You really may not want to have sex on a particular evening; you may not care that you didn't have an orgasm this time; you may be trying to tell him what feels good and what doesn't. Most men have a very hard time communicating verbally during sex. Some don't like to talk because they're afraid that a pause for conversation will cause them to lose that erection they've worked so hard for. They need to learn that a little detumescence never hurt anybody as long as it springs back up when needed. The nonverbal approach can be a real inhibitor to good sex. Talking during sex, and not just about the sex, helps relax you both, which enhances the experience. Share a laugh—this is not a funeral. Sexy talk can also be a real stimulant.

Myth 11. Good sex is spontaneous.
This is true only in the movies—and it only looks that way because it's been carefully scripted and rehearsed. Planning sex can increase anticipation, not to mention the likelihood that it will actually happen. If you decline sex, offer an alternative plan. "Not tonight, honey, I'm tired" can easily be followed by "See you in the morning." Of course there's nothing wrong with spontaneity; it can do a lot to rev up a relationship. It's only a problem when couples assume that all or even most sex should follow a sudden rush of desire.

Myth 12. Real men don't have sexual problems.
Many men assume that admitting a problem makes them less masculine and

less desirable. A man can cover up most health problems for a long time; he doesn't have to admit that he's having chest pains climbing stairs or that his knee hurts. Sexual problems are not so easy to hide from you. His only option is to avoid sex. If at all possible, don't let him avoid the problem or the sex. What he doesn't understand—and what you can help him understand—is that having a problem doesn't make him less a man in your eyes. Indeed, it may have the opposite effect. Admitting to a problem can humanize a man— not to mention make it possible to solve it.

Communicating About Sex

In helping a man break through most of these myths, the key is opening up the communication. Several times a year Ruth Jacobowitz, medical journalist and author of *150 Most-Asked Questions About Midlife Sex, Love, and Intimacy,* and I give seminars to groups of middle-age couples interested in improving their relationships. Even these couples, who strongly desire to improve their lives, have a difficult time talking about what bothers them.

Ruth and I often ask the group very direct questions. I might ask for a show of hands of people who think their sex life is better now than it was at age thirty. Ruth might ask the women in the audience whether their doctors have asked them if they're sexually satisfied. Quite often the answers to those sorts of questions surprise the audience and even the partners of those responding.

There are many questions that partners should be asking each other about their sex lives. How and when do you ask them? First and foremost, Ruth says, "Not in bed." She offers a suggestion from June Reinisch, Ph.D., that the car is a far better place. To avoid putting him on the defensive when you ask questions, don't imply there are problems. Instead, try to communicate positively about solutions. If he's having a problem with erections, express concern for his condition and urge him to talk to a doctor about it. If his behavior in bed isn't working for you, don't tell him what you don't want; tell him what you would like.

When you open up communication, the first step is the most difficult. The next step and the ones that follow are easier. You'll find that the impossible has become possible: Men can talk. The rewards are far more than resolving the issues at hand. The act of communicating is the best aphrodisiac in the world.

How to Fire Things Up

Despite all the sexual innuendoes in the media and advertising, most of everyday life isn't very sexy. It's filled with appointments to keep, deadlines to be met, shopping to be done, and bills to be paid. In the fog of daily obligations, your flame grows dim. Don't assume that it has gone out, though. Most of the time it just needs a little attention. Here are some suggestions:

• **Make a date.** Plan ahead for time together. Whether it's a special dinner out (or in) or a movie, discuss it well in advance so you both have plenty of time to anticipate the time together. Whatever you choose, be sure you won't be interrupted.

• **Exercise together.** Moderate exercise will boost both your sex drives. Also, it can be stimulating to do something intensely physical together—and in public, too!

• **You know what they say about variety.** Try a different room or even no room at all. Suggest a new position or just a different time of day for sex. The occasional surprise can reinvigorate the more usual get-togethers.

• **Bathe together more often.** The shower or tub doesn't have to be a scene for sex or even necessarily a prelude. The simple act of being together naked and helping each other wash builds familiarity and intimacy. It's another way of getting to know each other better. (And while you're there, you can do those partner-exams described in chapter 5.)

• **Be attuned to daily cycles.** Hormone levels vary throughout the day. For men, testosterone levels usually peak in early morning, shortly after dawn. That's also the time when the stress of the day is the farthest behind him—if you catch him before he has time to start worrying about the day to come. With a little cooperation you can make the day less stressful for both of you.

• **Ask what he likes and offer it on occasion.** There is no typical man when it comes to what's sexy, but just about every man has some preference. It could be anything from black lace to flannel nightgowns to nothing at all. Books or videos work for some and not for others. Let each other know what you like, and work together to see that each of you gets it.

• **Laugh together.** A funny movie or comedian can have a surprisingly sexy effect. When you share something joyous together, it can only lead to further sharing. An uproariously good time in bed is a logical outcome.

Which brings me to the last thing I like to tell men about sex: Lighten up! Sex isn't serious business; it's not work; and it's not the end of the world. Women in general are better at maintaining a light attitude about sex, and I sure hope some of your good humor will rub off on him. You may not convince him that sex is funny, but with any luck he'll at least decide it's fun.

15

These Things Happen

It might seem baffling, even impossible, that a readily treatable medical problem can break up an otherwise happy marriage, but I have seen it happen. The problem is flagging erections. A pattern of failures, and sometimes even one occurrence, can start a chain of psychological and emotional problems that end in divorce.

Jeff and his ex-wife are a good example. By the time he came to see me, it was already too late for their marriage. Jeff was trying to bounce back from the divorce and had decided (finally!) to see whether there was help for his erection problem. As we talked, he told me that his first failure had been more than six years ago and that the problem had grown worse. He had begun to avoid sexual situations—even gestures, such as hugging or holding hands, that could lead to sexual situations—because he was afraid he would fail. He and Sally had grown distant, and she came to suspect that there was someone else. After five years of this, she moved out and filed the papers.

Jeff was in his mid-forties at the time, an age when many men experience an erection problem occasionally. Moreover, he was at least twenty pounds overweight, which increases the probability. So I wasn't surprised that he'd had some problems. Then I noticed on his chart that he was taking blood pressure medication. I asked him when he had started taking the medicine, and he told me it was six years ago. I told him gently that the medicine could have caused that initial failure and that anxiety over a repeat performance made it more likely that he would fail again and again. The prescription for the blood pressure medicine ended up being a prescription for divorce. Working with his primary care doctor, we switched Jeff's medication, and his erections returned. To be honest, I don't know if Jeff and his ex had other problems that would have torn them apart anyway—he was a mighty unhappy guy when I met him—but I know for certain that his avoidable sexual troubles didn't help.

Erection problems are extremely common. There are 15 to 20 million American men who occasionally have trouble getting or maintaining an erection sufficient for their and their partner's mutual satisfaction. Doctors use the term erectile dysfunction (ED) for a problem that is occasional, one time, or always. Including their partners, who can be just as devastated, 40 million Americans, nearly one in four, have a potency problem.

And, indeed, men don't suffer alone. In a recent survey by the Impotence Institute of America, women whose partners were having trouble expressed frustration (41 percent), disappointment (29 percent), and rejection (18 percent). Almost 40 percent felt some responsibility for the problem. Almost two-thirds of the women were unaware of treatment options. Looking into the future, women over fifty expected to stay sexually active into their eighties, but half of them will have partners with erection problems by the time they are seventy.

There are other erection problems besides a soft penis, too. Premature ejaculation can be at least as frustrating, and penile curvature (Peyronie's disease) can make intercourse impossible. You need to know why these things happen, how they can be prevented, and what can be done. Above all, you need to know that it's not your fault.

So Many Possibilities

As you learned in chapter 13, "Men Unzipped," an erection is a complex process—so complicated that you could easily have wondered why it is usually dependable. In fact, there are numerous opportunities for trouble. Nevertheless, I say without hesitation that modern medicine can give an erection to any man who wants one.

The underlying cause of ED has to be discovered so that the approach can be matched to the problem. A treatment that would be a godsend for some couples would be useless or even harmful for others. To offer a specific example, a penile implant will give any man an erection—no matter the source of the problem—but there's no retreat since it replaces normal tissues. It should be a couple's last resort, not the first attempt at a solution. If a doctor says, "No erections? How about an implant?" try another doctor.

As recently as fifteen years ago most doctors agreed with Masters and

Johnson that 90 percent of failed or weak erections had psychological causes. They thought most of the rest of the guys just needed a shot of testosterone to get going. Fortunately, we've come a long way. Even Masters and Johnson have changed their minds. Today, according to the Impotence Institute of America, ED has a physiological component about 85 percent of the time, and usually the physical problem is not a lack of hormones.

On the other hand, *every* man who has an erection problem, no matter the source, also has a psychological problem. The physiology of an erection can't be separated from the psychology of an erection (unless you're willing to use a penile implant to solve the problem). Nature has equipped the male penis with a marvelous defense mechanism. When a man with an erection is threatened, the resulting rush of adrenaline almost immediately makes him flaccid. That's a great idea if he's trying to escape from a grizzly bear; an erection would only get in the way. Unfortunately, the same reaction occurs when the threat is not physical but emotional. If a man worries about whether he's going to have an erection, adrenaline may make sure he doesn't.

As was the case with Jeff, whose problem I described at the beginning of this chapter, a physiological problem often develops into an emotional one. A side effect of blood pressure medication may have started his erection problems, but Jeff could probably have had erections anyway if it weren't for his anxiety about performing with his wife. The emotions that a man and a woman experience when his penis won't rise can get in the way of a solution. Together the couple needs to work with a counselor to fully understand performance anxiety and how to combat it, and they should seek additional help if they're unsuccessful.

Besides blood pressure medication, what other health problems can get in the way of an erection? Probably the most common cause of ED is hardening or narrowing of the arteries that supply blood to the penis. That's right, it's the same atherosclerosis that can lead to a heart attack or stroke. When the clogged arteries lead to the penis, they reduce its ability to become erect.

Since a man with clogged arteries in one part of his body is likely to have them elsewhere, too, heart disease and erection problems often go together. In one study of men with heart disease, the more vessels were clogged in the heart, the greater and more frequent the sexual problems. Men with advanced heart disease had half as many erections as men with the least clogged arteries; their erections were also less than half as firm, and they had nearly twice the trouble achieving them. At the St. Louis Veterans Administration Hospital, over a quarter of men who seek help for ED related to a circulatory problem have a heart attack or stroke within three years. In comparison, fewer than 5 percent of men with adequate penile blood flow had a heart attack or stroke during that time. One study just published found that men who have more orgasms live longer. The question is, do orgasms extend life, or do men who have healthy bodies have more orgasms? The studies at the VA in St. Louis suggest the latter.

If inflow problems prevent a penis from fully inflating, the blood vessels and lacunae (lakes) inside the penis become stiff and plaque-coated, too. They can no longer expand and trap blood in the penis. Inflow problems lead to outflow problems. The arteries supplying the penis may clear somewhat if a man stops smoking, cleans up his diet, and takes up exercise, but there's no evidence that the deterioration to the tissues in the penis can be reversed.

After circulatory problems (and contributing to them, too), the second most common cause of impotence is smoking. A study reported in the *Journal of Epidemiology* found that otherwise healthy men aged thirty-one to forty-nine who smoke have one and a half times as many erection problems as those who don't. Among all men seeking help for ED, various studies have found that between 50 and 81 percent were current or former smokers. Nicotine constricts blood vessels, including those that supply the penis with blood. Smoking two high-nicotine cigarettes will measurably soften an erection.

Diabetes can play havoc with potency. Not only does it contribute to circulatory problems, but nerve damage (diabetic neuropathy) can disrupt the signals that initiate or maintain erections.

Some medications can profoundly affect a man's ability to become erect. Besides blood pressure medications such as the one Jeff took, oral drugs for diabetes, ulcer and irritable bowel syndrome treatments, some antidepressants, and some heart medications affect potency. The full list of drugs that have been implicated in ED is pages long, so it's always worth checking with your man's doctor or pharmacist if he has erection troubles while taking a medication. And don't forget that self-administered drug—alcohol. The stories of drinking men who had the interest but not the ability are legion.

Penile fractures can damage the chambers of the penis, producing leaks that prevent the chambers from inflating properly. The arteries and nerves that serve the penis (located behind the scrotum in the perineum) can be damaged by a blow to the pelvis or repeated minor trauma. One of my patients ran afoul of a fence he tried to leap over, and I've also seen long-distance bicyclists with erection problems. (Numbness of the penis during cycling is a warning sign. If your guy experiences it, he should change seats, alter his riding position, or reduce his mileage.)

Other health problems can cause potency problems, too. The majority of men with the neurological disorder multiple sclerosis have sexual problems. Strokes, nerve damage from alcoholism, paralysis from accidents, Parkinson's disease, surgery (especially prostate surgery, which we'll talk more about in chapter 20), and even spinal disk problems can cause ED.

Finally, some potency problems are purely psychological, especially among younger guys. Often men who are having a mental problem with erections have grown up with the *Playboy* mentality and expect their penises to rise on command. Therapy can be very helpful for such men, but a temporary medicine may help boost confidence. Sometimes it takes only a few successes to get a man beyond his anxiety.

Diagnosing ED

We urologists, the specialists who diagnose and treat impotence, have an impressive array of equipment to test for different causes of a potency problem, but most of it usually isn't needed. Your partner (and you) will begin by talking with the doctor about what's happened. The urologist should review all the medications your partner has been taking, ask about his drinking habits, and request a full medical history (including events that may seem unconnected to the problem). Your partner should then have a blood pressure test, a testicle exam (for cancer and for shriveling, which could be caused by hormone problems), and a prostate exam (including PSA, if appropriate). It's also a a good idea to have a blood test that measures both total and free testosterone. Though low hormone levels are rarely the cause of erection problems (only about 5 percent of the time at the Male Health Institute), the blood test can also turn up other problems, such as diabetes, high cholesterol, and thyroid problems. (It's an opportunity to check for conditions that men otherwise might ignore. Each month I discover that two or three men with erection problems also have diabetes. What's the point of fixing an erection problem if the guy won't live long enough to enjoy it because of the preventable effects of diabetes, heart disease, or hypertension?)

I ask every man who sees me for a potency problem also to talk to a psychologist with whom I practice, although some refuse. As I've already pointed out, most potency problems are not psychological at their roots, but 100 percent of men with potency problems have an emotional problem as a result. If at all possible, you should be there, too. Not only is ED a couple's disease, but it usually takes both partners working together to solve the problem.

Many urologists have found a test called an erection injection to be one of the most effective tools in diagnosing potency problems that don't respond to Viagra. I inject a substance that occurs naturally in the body, called prostaglandin E1, through a *tiny* needle (next to no pain). PgE1 relaxes the smooth muscles in the penis to produce an erection in most men within ten minutes. The quality of that erection (on a one-to-ten scale) tells a lot about inflow problems, and the length of time it lasts tells a lot about outflow problems. Many guys, however, get so anxious at the thought of a needle and are so distracted by the medical office environment, with constant interruptions, that not even PgE1 will overcome the adrenaline racing through their bodies. After some instruction on the use of the injections, a little field-testing at home can be helpful.

Back in chapter 5, "Flashing Red Lights," I described the postage stamp test, a self-test to show whether a man is having normal erections at night while he sleeps. Doctors have more sophisticated tools to do the same job. A snap gauge, which consists of several strings of various strengths, gives more than a yes-or-no idea of nighttime activity. There are also electronic recording devices (nocturnal penile tumescence, or NPT) to accomplish this, but the cost is justified by the gain in information in very few cases.

When a man turns out to have a blood flow problem, the urologist may perform some additional tests to figure out the exact cause. Doppler ultrasound allows us to measure the blood flow into the penis and the size of the arteries; by giving an erection injection, we can see if the flow increases to certain levels and also if there are leaks. Another test called dynamic infusion cavernosometry and cavernosography (DICC), done at a hospital on an outpatient basis, shows the exact blood pressure in the penis, the rate of flow in and out, and which vessels might be leaking. Most men won't ever need DICC, but no man should have vascular surgery or an implant without it.

Depending on your man's age and physical condition, he might have some tests to check nerve function. Some of these are as simple as pin pricks or response to a vibrating tuning fork. The bulbocavernosal reflex, which contracts the rectum when the head of the penis is squeezed—I assure men I'm not getting fresh—is another clue to proper nerve operation. Biothesiometry, in which a vibration is applied to the penis by a sort of electrical tuning fork, measures the threshold of sensation, which is an important part of getting an erection. The doctor may also check the pulse and blood pressure in the penis, although there are differences of opinion over the accuracy of such measurements. At the same time the doctor should examine the penis for plaques that may be a sign of Peyronie's disease (more about that shortly).

Solving Potency Problems

Back in the sixties there were hormones. The implant came along in the seventies. Today there are dozens of options for solving potency problems. As you and your partner consider them, remember:

• You, the woman, should be included every step of the way; this is a plural "you" problem.

• Every problem can be treated; impotence is not something you two have to live with.

• Impotence often has multiple causes, and it's often not necessary to eliminate all them. The penis can be like a set of scales weighed down by a collection of things. If he can eliminate a few, the balance will shift, and up it will pop.

• There are always treatment *options*; there is never only one best treatment. The most sensible approach is to try the simplest, least invasive techniques first.

The following treatments are listed roughly in order of their ease, expense, and reversibility.

Oral Medications

If you missed 1998's big news on treatment for erectile dysfunction, you and yours must have been holed up on some desert island. Pfizer's release of Viagra has caused quite a stir—in the press and in homes—and deservedly so. At the risk of seeming overly enthusiastic, it's probably the most important development in the treatment of erection problems since I began practicing medicine. Nonetheless, Viagra isn't for everyone, it's not a substitute for solving the problem that caused the erection problem in the first place, and it doesn't rule out other therapies. Before Viagra enters your relationship, you and your partner need to understand what it will and won't do, and how it might affect your lives.

First of all, Viagra is quite effective. Clinical studies have found that 70 to 80 percent of men who take it see a significant improvement in their erections, and our experience at the Male Health Institute has been even better. It is slightly less effective for men whose erectile dysfunction results from diabetes, prostate-cancer surgery, or spinal-cord injury, but it still helps many of them achieve an erection. Viagra does absolutely nothing, however, to increase the desire for an erection or to delay ejaculation. It is not an aphrodisiac. Nor if a man is functioning normally will it any way enhance his performance. A short look into how it works will show why.

If you recall our discussion of how an erection occurs, you may remember that nitric oxide triggers the release of some funny-sounding enzymes and chemicals in penile smooth-muscle cells. One of those, cGMP, reduces calcium concentrations in the cells, so the cells can relax. The counterpart of cGMP, called 5 phosphodiesterase enzyme (PDE5), breaks down cGMP. Viagra works by blocking the action of PDE5, enhancing natural erections, so it will do nothing unless there's stimulation to produce the nitric oxide and cGMP in the first place.

Some men should absolutely not take Viagra. First on the list are those who are taking nitrate-based medications (nitroglycerin, for example) for angina or high blood pressure. The combination can be deadly. Some of the deaths reported among Viagra users are no doubt attributable to nitrates, but it's worth noting that one in 50,000 men who do not take Viagra have heart attacks during sex. When a seventy-year-old man gets the erection of a thirty-year-old and acts like a twenty-year-old, things can happen. Dosages need to be adjusted for men who are taking erythromycin (an antibiotic), cimetidine (an antiulcer medication), ketoconazole (an antifungal), and rifampin (for tuberculosis). Taking Viagra with food reduces or eliminates its effectiveness. Viagra's side effects are mainly minor but worth noting. Among the 10 percent of men who experience a side effect, 16 percent have headache, 10 percent facial flushing, 7 percent indigestion, 4 percent nasal congestion, 2 percent dizziness, and 3 percent vision abnormalities (mainly color shifts). Doses over 100 milligrams significantly increase these side effects without being more effective. More is not better.

One of my biggest concerns about widespread, indiscriminate use of Viagra is that it may become a substitute for concern about and treatment of the source of the erection problem. Most men who have a problem getting or maintaining an erection also have an underlying physical problem that may threaten their life. Heart disease and diabetes are two examples. Viagra might give a man with one of these diseases erections, but he may not be around long to enjoy them, unless they are treated.

A further potential problem is a sort of dependency on the drug. Although there is no physical dependency, Viagra must be taken an hour before sex. How does a man know if or when he no longer needs the drug to achieve an erection?

Viagra can also disrupt established marital patterns. Stories of men who discover Viagra and quickly become unfaithful are already appearing. Men like to think that having an erection will solve any marital problem, but you know better! Intercourse is a natural part of a fulfilling relationship, but it's not the basis of one.

The drug yohimbine, made from the bark of an African tree called yohimbe, has been touted for decades for its enhancement of both sexual desire and erections. Until recently, however, scientific research about yohimbine's effectiveness was inconsistent. Some studies reported a positive effect; others found no benefit beyond a placebo effect. In late 1997 investigators at the University of Exeter in England reviewed the studies available, picked seven they judged of sufficient quality, and "meta-analyzed" their results. This work showed a clear benefit to yohimbine over a placebo, especially for younger men.

Yohimbine causes few side effects in most people (some have occasional jitters or increased blood pressure), and it's inexpensive. If you want to try it, use the prescription variety; over-the-counter yohimbine products have inconsistent dosages and are no less expensive than prescription preparations. The only real disadvantages to yohimbine is that he'll need to remember to take it three times a day and that improvement doesn't usually occur for two to six weeks.

A couple of years ago I prescribed yohimbine for a man who'd been having erection difficulties. He returned after two months and reported that he had had sex forty-seven times in the previous three weeks. Whether yohimbine's effect is psychological (placebo) or physiological, its influence was powerful for that guy.

In the past year, two other oral medications have shown some promise in clinical trials. Apomorphine, placed under the tongue to be absorbed, works on the brain. In one trial it enabled about 60 percent of men with psychological impotence to achieve erections half the time. Side effects are limited to nausea in about 11 percent of men, with occasional vomiting and hiccups. (Stronger injected doses of apomorphine have been used to induce vomiting, so this isn't surprising.) Assuming that trials continue to be positive, apomorphine might become available during 1999.

Phentolamine is a compound used routinely in three-part erection injections, but an oral medication is new. It works by dilating blood vessels, which appears to improve erections in about 40 to 50 percent of men who take it. Like the other two oral drugs, phentolamine has no effect on libido. It works in conjunction with normal sexual stimulation between twenty and sixty minutes after it is taken. Phentolamine might become available as early as late 1998.

The whole area of oral medications for ED is really new, and we have a lot to learn about how they work and what works best. It may be that some drugs work best in combination, but we just don't know. Keep an eye open for developments.

Hormone Supplements

I discuss supplementation of testosterone and other hormones in detail in chapter 21, "Guy Troubles." However, hormone supplements are rarely the answer. Among my patients, low hormone levels are the cause of potency problems only about 5 percent of the time. Also, supplements can increase the risk of certain cancers. At the Male Health Institute we treated a man who had been given testosterone shots by another doctor for two years. The shots did nothing to solve his potency problem. He came to us because he was having difficulty urinating. We found very advanced prostate cancer.

Pelvic Floor Biofeedback

Although the muscles *inside* the penis must relax in order for a man to have an erection, consciously tensing up the muscles that contract when he ejaculates (some outside the penis, some inside) may help erections. We've known for some time that when the ischiocavernosus (IC) and bulbocavernosus (BC) muscles contract, blood pressure inside the penis increases significantly, stiffening the erection. Usually these muscles operate without any conscious thought, but it occurred to a group of Belgian researchers that men might be taught to use and strengthen the IC muscle to improve erections that were not stiff enough for intercourse.

We've experimented with this technique at the Male Health Institute. The exercise is similar to the one known as Kegels that women do to strengthen the muscles of the pelvic floor. Men can be taught to contract the proper muscles, too. The Belgians used electrical stimulation to contract the IC muscle so that the men could feel the proper muscles contract. Biofeedback sensors can also be used.

In the Belgian study, the goal was to improve the rigidity of men's erections. After four months of pelvic exercise training, 69 out of 155 men were cured, and another 42 had improved. Results at my clinic have not been quite as encouraging, but I think the approach is worth pursuing further because it is so noninvasive and because a fitter pelvic floor benefits men as well as women. I'll describe Kegel exercises further in chapter 20.

Vacuum Devices

Next to oral medications a vacuum device is the least invasive treatment for ED, though not necessarily the least expensive or obtrusive. A vacuum pump is a plastic cylinder that fits snugly over the penis and is sealed to the body with petroleum jelly. Some are pumped manually; others are battery operated. Either way, the device produces negative pressure around the penis, which causes blood to flow in and produce an erection. Once the erection is established, an elastic ring can be slipped onto the base of the penis to hold blood in so the tube can be removed.

If a vacuum device is used properly—instruction is important—it will produce an erection for just about any man. (They have been used successfully on paralyzed men who have no sensation in their penis.) One drawback may be a hinge effect if the portion of the penis inside the body is not as rigid as the portion outside (because the constriction ring at the base is maintaining the erection). The restriction of blood flow may make the penis's skin feel colder than usual, again because the blood flow is restricted. The constriction ring can cause damage if left on longer than thirty minutes. Like learning to roller-skate, learning to use a vacuum device takes practice, and I recommend that men try it ahead of time.

Despite these minor disadvantages, vacuum devices are a good solution for many men and their partners. Although they require some planning and preparing for sex, they work well and have no side effects. Some men discover that after using a vacuum device for a while, they're able to get an erection without the device. This could be because of the restorative effects of pulling fresh, oxygenated blood into the penis or because of the confidence built up by knowing they can have an erection. It's probably a combination of the two.

Your spouse should obtain his vacuum device through his doctor to be sure he gets a high-quality device that's the right size and also gets proper instruction (videos are available). The Food and Drug Administration recently approved over-the-counter sales, but not all brands are available that way, and the right fit and instruction are crucial. He can expect to pay between $200 and $400, depending on bells and whistles, but some urologists will be willing to lend him one. The Male Health Institute has one of the largest collections in Texas. I encourage men with erection problems that don't respond to Viagra to at least give a vacuum device a try. I've started taking a deposit when men check one out at the Institute; too many have worked so well that they didn't come back!

Not every couple can accept the fact that a vacuum device requires either planning or a pause in sexual activity, but many find it a perfectly satisfactory and safe way to enjoy sex again. One man was so enthusiastic about the unit we lent him that he refused to return it until his prescription-ordered vacuum device arrived. Another man's wife makes sure he doesn't pack the vacuum device when he travels—unless she's going along!

Urethral Inserts

The MUSE system for administering prostaglandin E1 (PgE1) was approved by the FDA in 1997. A small plastic plunger places a pellet of Alprostadil (a type of PgE1) about the size of a grain of rice inside the urethra, where it's absorbed into the corpora cavernosum. About one-third of impotent men are able to have intercourse with this treatment. Restriction bands help further. The side effects are usually minor; the most common are mild penile pain (about 11 percent) and dizziness (about 3 percent). The first insertion should be in a medical office, to determine proper dosage, manage side effects, and develop proper technique, which is crucial. Then he's on his own.

Acceptance of inserts has been almost universal at my clinic, as an alternative to injections. Some men have a powerful aversion to needles in that neighborhood. If oral approaches fail and a vacuum device isn't appealing, inserts are definitely worth a try. They may also be effective in combination with other methods such as Viagra.

Erection Injections

About 85 percent of all men with potency problems, regardless of their origin, respond to an injection of prostaglandin E1 or a combination of prostaglandin E1, papaverine, and phentolamine (often called trimix). All these drugs relax the smooth muscle in the penis. The needle is the tiniest made, and it is inserted in an area with very few nerve endings. Although any sensible man would be apprehensive before his first injection, most find that it's not uncomfortable. Giving yourself a shot requires some instruction, but it's not difficult. Within five to ten minutes he gets a stiff erection that lasts thirty to sixty minutes. Even after ejaculation the erection may not go away until the drug fades. Once a man has had his first injection in the office, it's not uncommon for him to ask for a gallon of the drug to go.

Only two of these drugs—prostaglandin E1 as a part of Caverject and EDEX—are approved by the FDA for erection injection, but all of the above-mentioned medications have been proved safe in other applications and have been used for almost ten years to create erections. A new compound, vasoactive intenstinal polypeptide (or VIP), has recently been approved. PgE1 is a naturally occurring compound in the body. The primary side effect, a burning sensation after injection, is caused by the acidity of the medicines. Buffering them with sodium bicarbonate appears to eliminate this problem. There have also been reports of scarring and nodules (Peyronie's disease) in about 7 percent of men, but mainly with papaverine used alone, which is out of favor in the medical community.

An erection that won't go away is always a risk with injections, especially early on when trying to establish the correct dosage. Any erection that lasts longer than two hours requires immediate medical attention to prevent damage to the penis.

Injections aren't for everyone, but many men find them a very acceptable way to get and maintain an erection. It's not unusual for a man without major physical problems to return to normal erections after using injections for a while.

One good example of a man satisfied with injection therapy is a fellow who came to me after emergency abdominal surgery had damaged the nerves that control erection. He'd been unable to have an erection for seven years and had simply given up on sex. In my office he responded immediately to prostaglandin E1, and his first comment to the nurse on hand was "How often can I use this stuff?" (The answer is, about three times a week.) He's now one of the strongest advocates around for erection injections, and at sixty-four he remarried. He passes along these comments; "I've been on injection therapy for three years. It is flawless, and there are no side effects for me. It's very, very easy to do. Within five or six minutes it's there, as big as I've ever had, and I know it's going to be there. It works."

Vascular Surgery

When other options fail, it's time to consider surgical correction. A few years ago many urologists and patients opted for vascular surgery, in which arteries and/or veins are rearranged or blocked off to solve inflow or outflow problems. Since then, doctors have learned that this isn't the right approach for most men. Typically, when a man has arterial problems, all his arteries, blood vessels, and the spongy tissue of the penis are affected, so patching a few vessels doesn't do the job. Even for ideal candidates—young men who have been injured and don't smoke—the success rate is only about 60 percent.

Vascular surgery is never the solution unless there are specific flow problems rather than a general inability to block outflow. Be very certain that the exact problem has been found, and get a second opinion before proceeding. This is a case where not just any urologist should be doing the work. Seek out an experienced, skilled surgeon at a university medical center or in a practice that specializes in potency treatments and vascular surgery.

After casting all that doubt on vascular surgery, I think it's worth mentioning that it can be very successful. I treated an eighteen-year-old man who came to me when considering marriage. He had never been able to have an erection and wanted to know if there was any way he could consummate his marriage if he were to go ahead. We were able to find specific vein leaks using DICC, he opted for surgery, and six weeks later he was married and able to function. I got a note from him two years later saying that everything was fine and that he and his wife had just had their first child.

Penile Implants

When a man can't or won't succeed with other treatments, an implant is the last resort. Of all the approaches, this one should be taken least lightly. Once he's had an implant, his chances of ever functionally normally without one are gone. An implant can be removed, but erections will be possible only with a vacuum device in some cases. One of the saddest things I see in my practice is a man who has had an implant that he didn't really need. Get at least a second opinion before considering an implant, and select the surgeon carefully. Ask about his or her experience and rate of success.

However, just because an implant is the last resort doesn't mean it's not a good one. About ten thousand penile implants are done each year—at least 250,000 men have had them since they were developed—and the majority of these men and their spouses are delighted with the result. It's not like being eighteen again, but it can make the difference between having and not having intercourse.

An implant does nothing but allow a man to have an erect penis. He will have the same sensation—good if it was so, not so good if it wasn't—and he will be able ejaculate normally if he was able to before. The device goes in the corpus cavernosa. It may be semirigid, meaning that it can be manually raised and lowered, or it may be inflated with a small squeeze bulb. The most sophisticated ones not only make the penis stiff but also increase penis length during inflation.

Penile prostheses have been around for more than twenty-five years. Dr. Brantley Scott of Houston pioneered the bionics for the first implant, but those early devices bear little resemblance to today's. Modern implants are easier to install and more effective. My first implant surgery took two and a half hours; today it takes only fifty minutes, requires only a four-inch incision, and is an outpatient procedure.

There are several different types of implants and a number of concerns. The materials are different from breast implants so there's no concern about silicone. Going into the concerns in detail is beyond the scope of this book, but I encourage you and your partner to study carefully, get a copy of a 1993 FDA report on implants, watch videos that are available, and talk to several doctors as well as to men who've had implants. As with any surgery, infection is possible. The implant may migrate or fail mechanically, or scar tissue may develop around it, causing problems. Also, once an implant is installed, natural erections will never be possible again even if the implant is removed.

Out of concern for potential problems with implants, I reviewed the situation of the more than one hundred men in whom I've installed them. Ninety-five percent said they were satisfied and would do it again, and 50 percent said they would go on national television to advocate penile implants. This degree of satisfaction is, I believe, the result of proper selection and education of the men so they knew what they were getting. A modern implant, when properly installed in the right patient, can work wonders. It restores a man's ability to enjoy a full relationship with his partner.

One patient at the Male Health Institute told me that he had willed his body to medical science after his death—all, that is, except his implant. He told me, "Doc, I want to be sure I have my implant with me when I get where I'm going."

Psychological Treatment

Counseling should be part of every ED treatment. There's no sense working on a penis as if it's not attached to a whole man who has fears, emotions, and worries. You need to explore those feelings with him and with a skilled, professional counselor. I'm not talking about psychoanalysis. Counseling for potency patients means understanding performance anxiety and figuring out how to control it, resolving marital issues on both sides, and treating any depression. Getting the penis to work is the easy part!

Premature Ejaculation

When is ejaculation premature? If it's defined as ejaculating within five minutes of beginning intercourse, 36 million American couples suffer from it.

(It's been estimated that the average act of intercourse lasts five minutes.) Many fewer couples would be affected under another common definition: *frequently* ejaculating unintentionally before or shortly after beginning intercourse. The only meaningful definition: Is ejaculation too premature for you and your partner's satisfaction?

Myths about Premature Ejaculation

Premature ejaculation does *not* happen for these reasons:
- Men get too excited to focus on bodily sensations.
- Men's early sexual experiences were in situations where hurrying was beneficial (such as in a car), so they learned a bad habit.
- Men are so concerned about their performance that they ignore their own sensations.
- Men feel guilty about enjoying sex or pleasure of any kind.
- Men are worried about maintaining their erection.
- Men have unresolved relationship issues.
- Men are under too much stress.

Common approaches that *won't* work:
- Long-term psychoanalysis
- Getting drunk
- Using one or more condoms
- Concentrating on something other than sex—such as one's bank balance—while having intercourse
- Biting one's cheek as a distraction
- Frequent masturbation
- Creams that numb the penis
- Testosterone injections
- Tranquilizers

The more men I treat for premature ejaculation (over three thousand so far), the more I'm convinced that it is a physical problem. During ejaculation the muscles surrounding the penis become active to expel semen. In men with premature ejaculation, these muscles are often hyperactive, heading too fast toward contraction. Also, research has shown that many men who ejaculate prematurely are more sensitive to vibration in the penis than other men.

Before a man begins treatment for premature ejaculation, it may be appropriate for him to talk to a psychologist about other conflicts that may be affecting his performance. It's not unusual for a man to imagine that he can solve his marital problems by lasting longer. Relationship problems always go deeper than that. Men also can have premature ejaculation problems related to impotence. Because they're so worried about losing an erection, they rush ejaculation.

These learned responses aren't easy to erase. Nonetheless, a leading expert in this field, Helen Singer Kaplan, found that premature ejaculation, though it often causes a great deal of emotional trauma, is rarely a psychological problem at the root. Although she was a psychiatrist, Dr. Kaplan didn't recommend intense psychological therapy to help men get control. Instead, she encouraged men and their partners to talk openly about the situation, perhaps in the presence of a counselor, and practice step-by-step methods for getting control.

The Squeeze Method

This approach was developed by Masters and Johnson. The partner stimulates the man's penis until he is close to ejaculating. He must learn to tell her when he's about to ejaculate, at which time she squeezes his penis with her hand hard enough to make him partially lose his erection. By wrapping the fingers around the penis just below the head, a squeeze will efficiently prevent ejaculation. The goal is for the man to become well enough aware of the sensations that he becomes trained to forestall his orgasm on his own. The technique progresses from manual stimulation to motionless intercourse with the woman on top, to her moving, and to both partners moving.

The Stop-Start Method

This approach was first used by Dr. James Stearn in 1955, and Dr. Kaplan and other therapists refined it considerably. Dr. Kaplan described the method in great detail in her book *PE: How to Overcome Premature Ejaculation*, but briefly here is what's involved. (Dr. Bernie Zilbergeld's book *The New Male Sexuality* also discusses techniques for solving premature ejaculation.)

Stop-start begins much like the squeeze method except that the woman just stops stimulating the man's penis when he asks her to—before the point of inevitability. As soon as he's certain he's under control, he asks her to begin rubbing again. This procedure is repeated three times before allowing ejaculation on the fourth. After the couple has repeated this two or three times a week and he has gained good control, stop-start with lubrication is introduced. After that has been mastered, intercourse with the woman on top and the man not moving can be attempted. Again he asks that she stop when he approaches the point of no return. That's followed by female-on-top intercourse with the man moving his hips, which is followed by stop-start, side-by-side intercourse. Finally, slowing down is substituted for stopping and starting.

Using this approach, Dr. Kaplan reported being able to cure 70 to 80 percent of her patients. In my own practice the success rate is not quite as high, largely because partners aren't always cooperative about performing all the steps and the results aren't always long lasting. A man can practice stop-start without a partner, but the effects go only so far. If both of you are willing to work diligently with Kaplan's techniques, you should give them a try. If they're a bit more than you bargained for, there are other options.

Biofeedback Therapy

Biofeedback can help a man become aware of the muscles that control ejaculation and learn how to control them. We've achieved significant success with this approach at the Male Health Institute, but it requires the use of a rectal plug and self-stimulation, which many men are reluctant to go through. A screen alerts a man to rising tension in his ejaculatory muscles, allowing him to anticipate and eventually control ejaculation. Unfortunately, the equipment and expertise needed for this approach are not widely available.

Pharmacological Therapy

The easiest way to halt premature ejaculation is to take advantage of a side effect of certain antidepressant medications: the tricyclic clomipramine (Anafranil) and two different selective seratonin reuptake inhibitors (SSRIs): fluoxetine (Prozac), and sertraline (Zoloft). All of these medications reduce libido and impair orgasm. Usually these side effects are seen as undesirable, but recent studies have looked at their more positive aspects for men who have problems with premature ejaculation.

Clomipramine appears to be the most effective at delaying ejaculation. In one trial, men with an average time of forty-six seconds until ejaculation during intercourse were able to extend that to five minutes, forty-five seconds. Among the SSRIs, sertraline showed the best performance at four minutes, sixteen seconds. The SSRIs as a group caused fewer undesirable side effects, such as drowsiness, dry mouth, and constipation. Another study of twenty-five couples found that clomipramine increased time to ejaculation by two and a half to five times, depending on dose. What's more, three women who had never experienced coital orgasm were able to, and women who often had coital orgasms increased their frequency. Most of my patients take one or two pills about two hours before intercourse; if it doesn't work, we try a different SSRI. Continuous medication, which can be expensive, is rarely necessary.

Whether medication is continuous or occasional, the benefits disappear if the medication is discontinued.

Penile Curvature: Peyronie's Disease

A decade ago I was on a campaign to bring impotence out of the closet. I knew that my patients represented only a tiny fraction of the men (and women) who actually suffered from the problem. Today, although only about 5 percent of men with potency problems are getting help, we're making real progress. Now I have a new campaign: to bring Peyronie's disease out of the closet.

Peyronie's disease causes a curved penis. No one knows how common it is. Some health officials have "guesstimated" that about 1 percent of men have it, but I think it's much more common. I see two or three men per day whose curvature has become severe enough to affect intercourse, and most of them had never heard of Peyronie's disease before entering my office.

Named after the French physician who first diagnosed the disorder back in 1743, Peyronie's disease has no known cause. It may occur when the penis does not heal normally after an injury caused by rough intercourse, constriction rings, self-injection therapy, or a blow. The problem starts as a small inflamed bump below the skin on the shaft of the penis. The bump expands to form a flat calcium deposit that's sometimes as large as a silver dollar.

Because the deposit is not flexible like the normal tissue of the penis, when a man with Peyronie's has an erection, his penis can't expand completely on one side. Most of the time it bends in a J shape, but I sometimes see a U or even a corkscrew. About one-third of men with Peyronie's have painful erections, and as many as 20 percent become impotent. They're often happy to hear that they don't have cancer.

Until very recently men with Peyronie's had few good options. We could suggest taking 400 international units of vitamin E twice a day or the drug colchicine. Neither oral approach was supported by scientific trials, but at worst they do no harm. We also recommended waiting before taking drastic action such as surgery. Peyronie's resolves itself in about 30 percent of cases, although a man's penis will never return to its former shape and size.

A couple of years ago, however, a new technique involving injection of the drug verapamil was developed by Laurence Levine at Rush–St. Luke's Medical Center in Chicago. Fifty of my patients have participated in trials of verapamil. About 60 percent enjoy significant reduction in curvature, and most have less pain. One sure sign that it helps is that the men were willing to undergo twelve injections of the medication into the penis, and some even asked for a second round of treatment.

Unfortunately, verapamil won't work for the many—I suspect most—men who don't seek help soon after noticing symptoms. Because verapamil reduces formation of the plaque, which takes up to a year and a half, it's too late for injections once the plaque has fully formed. If you've noticed a significant new turn in his penis—even a normal penis isn't perfectly straight—be sure he sees a knowledgeable urologist right away.

When Peyronie's disease progresses to the point where intercourse becomes impossible, and verapamil and patience haven't worked, surgical correction can be done. The simplest approach is to shorten the long side by removing a wedge, called plication, or a derivation of plication called the Nesbitt procedure. This does shorten the penis about an inch, but complications are rare, including leaking veins (which can cause impotence). For more severe curvature it may be necessary to cut the plaque and apply a skin graft. Unfortunately, in this case impotence is common (rates as high as 70 percent in some reports), and the skin may be numb if nerves are damaged. Standard impotence therapies such as vacuum devices, urethral inserts, or injections may take care of that. And when everything else fails, there's always the ever-reliable last resort—the penile implant.

Clearly, although we're making progress in treating Peyronie's disease, we can't yet claim to have a good cure. Fortunately, severe curvatures are relatively rare. My patient Paul is more typical. At fifty-four, Paul has had Peyronie's for seven years. His bend isn't severe enough to prevent intercourse, he can still get erections, and he and his partner are still enjoying sex. He'd like to have a straight penis, and we've discussed the alternatives and the risks involved. Together, he and his wife have decided that his condition is something they can live with.

16

"Let's Not Use a Condom Just This Once"

I n my professional experience, most people think that sexually transmitted diseases (STDs) happen to *other* people, people who are wild, careless, or degenerate. Most of us, myself included, were taught that in our youth.

If only "others" get STDs, there are a heck of a lot of "others." At least a quarter of all American adults have an incurable sexually transmitted disease. About 55 million carry an STD right now, and 12 million are newly infected each year. More than one in five Americans has genital herpes, and genital warts aren't far behind. I tell men that when they go to a baseball game, the odds are even that there's a person with an STD within arm's length. The same is true at a play or a PTA meeting.

Very few people have a solid understanding of how common STDs are and how likely infection is. What's worse, many of today's most devastating STDs cannot be cured! The aftermath of a one-night stand can last a lifetime—and in the case of HIV infection, a drastically shortened one.

A woman's risk is even greater than a man's. For example, although 21.9 percent of *people* have herpes, 25.6 percent of *women* have it, as opposed to 17.8 percent of men. A woman is twice as likely as a man to contract one of several types of STDs from a single encounter. Also, some STDs cause obvious symptoms in men but not in women, so a woman may not know she needs treatment. Some STDs cause more health problems for women than for men. Chlamydia has minimal effects on men but may be responsible for 15 percent of infertility in women.

You may be thinking that *you* don't have anything to worry about because you have a monogamous relationship with a faithful man. Maybe. How long have you two been together? As a general rule, at least a year of monogamy is necessary to rule out the appearance of most diseases, but some take considerably longer to show up. Some STDs may not have any symptoms, so he may not know he has one and can transmit it. You may not know you have one, either. Perhaps you've both had tests for HIV if there was any risk. That's smart, but it doesn't rule out other possibilities that it's not practical to test for.

It isn't simple to make decisions about your risks of STDs, about the appropriate precautions, or about what to do if one crops up in your life. Even those of us who have done everything we can to rule out risk in our lives have sons and daughters to worry about. AIDS is now the number one killer of men between the ages of twenty-five and forty-four, and many of them were infected when they were carefree teenagers.

An Alphabetical Rogue's Gallery

The list of foreign-sounding villains that lie in wait looks scary, and it should, but if you and yours learn about STDs and take precautions, they don't have to be a part of your life. Make decisions based on the facts, and don't ignore the possibilities. So let's take a look at the major STDs and talk about how they could affect you and your man.

AIDS

Acquired immune deficiency syndrome, caused by human immunodeficiency virus (HIV), is first not just in alphabetical order but also among most people's concerns. And rightfully so. Although HIV infection isn't as common as many other STDs (there are about forty thousand new cases each year in the United States), it's the only STD that is almost certainly fatal. (Drug combinations have greatly extended and improved the lives of AIDS patients, but the virus has yet to be halted entirely.)

Since the beginning of the AIDS epidemic in the early 1980s, most women haven't worried much about themselves. AIDs was associated with homosexual contact between men or intravenous drug use. Now the picture is changing. Although male homosexual contact and IV drug use remain the behaviors that lead most often to AIDS, heterosexual contact is the fastest growing cause; among women it accounted for more than half of new cases with a known cause between July 1996 and June 1997. Women are also becoming a larger part of the mortality statistics. As recently as 1990, only 2,800 women died of AIDS; by 1995 the number had jumped to 7,200.

HIV infection is transmitted through blood, semen, and vaginal secretions. It can be passed from mother to fetus and through breast milk. It is not transmitted through saliva, urine, feces, tears, or sweat. The infection may remain latent for years before causing symptoms, but laboratory tests will almost always reveal its presence, although not until six months after infection.

If you and your guy have settled into a monogamous relationship within the last year and have any reason to think that either of you has been exposed to HIV, tests are a good idea. Reasons to suspect that you may have been exposed are numerous: unprotected sex with anyone of undetermined status, multiple sex partners, intravenous drug use, and so on. Chances are that the tests will put your minds at rest. Until HIV is ruled out, use a combination of condoms and spermicide. Statisticians have shown that you're safer having protected sex with a person with HIV than having unprotected sex with someone whose HIV status is unknown.

Candidiasis (Yeast Infection)

This fungal infection is familiar to many women and largely unknown to men. Nonetheless, a man can harbor the fungi and pass them back to his female partner, causing a rebound infection. (By the way, only rarely have I found evidence of fungi in men who are circumcised.) Most men (except those with diabetes or an immune system problem) experience only a mild rash, but women have intense itching, burning, and redness in the vaginal area; a white discharge; and possibly pain during intercourse. If you have these symptoms, see your doctor for a test and prescription medication. If you've had a yeast infection before and are absolutely certain it's the same thing it's safe to use over-the-counter medications.

If you keep getting fungal infections over and over again, consider using condoms until over-the-counter antifungal creams have absolutely eradicated any evidence of fungus in both of you.

Chancroid

Chancroid is a bacterial infection that develops four to fourteen days after exposure. Pustular, irregular, usually painful craters develop rapidly. Chancroid can produce whole-body symptoms, including fever and swollen lymph nodes. Fortunately, antibiotics are usually effective.

Chancroid is rare in the United States today. Fewer than a thousand cases were reported in 1995. As recently as 1987 the rates were nearly ten times higher, and they remain much higher in tropical countries. Condoms are quite effective at preventing the spread of this infection.

Chlamydia

A relative newcomer, chlamydia bacterial infection only made the Centers for Disease Control (CDC) charts in 1984. Since then, however, it has become one of the most commonly reported STDs; the CDC estimates that there are about 4 million new cases each year. About a quarter of men and three-quarters of women who get chlamydia never develop symptoms, but it remains contagious at all times. Possible symptoms are a burning sensation during urination, a clear or creamy discharge from the vagina or the tip of the penis, and sometimes itching seven to twenty-eight days after exposure.

Untreated chlamydia can cause pelvic inflammatory disease in women, which can lead to sterility or life-threatening tubal pregnancy. A recently suggested link between chlamydia and cervical cancer deserves further study. Pregnant women may pass it to their babies. In men it can cause sterility, urethral problems, prostatitis, and epididymitis.

Should either of you be diagnosed with chlamydia, you both should be treated with antibiotics, and you should use condoms until the course of drugs is finished.

Condyloma

Condyloma is a viral wart that occurs on the genitals or anus. There are more than 70 forms of human papillomavirus (HPV). Some produce visible warts (they aren't the type of warts that appear on hands or feet). Others, the most dangerous types, are invisible unless the doctor enhances them with a stain. After exposure, warts don't show up for one to three months or even a lot longer.

Condyloma may be much more common than doctors have thought; in one survey almost half of college women had it. It's estimated that more than 4 million Americans have active condyloma and that 10 to 20 percent of the population carry the virus. One reason HPV is so prevalent is its efficient transmission. There is a two-thirds chance of getting it from one encounter. Symptoms need not be present for infection to occur.

The greatest concern with HPV is the association between some forms and both cervical and penile cancer. Specifically, types 16 and 18 of HPV are frequently found in biopsies of cervical cancers. (There are tests to identify HPV type, but they're expensive.) A 1996 study in Spain found that if a woman's husband had HPV 16 on his penis, her risk of cervical cancer was increased by nine times. (Beyond HPV, her risk was also increased by her husband's other sexual behaviors: first intercourse at an early age [3.2 times], more than twenty sexual partners [11 times], sex with prostitutes [8 times], or chlamydia [2.6 times]. Clearly, a man's behavior can have quite an effect on a woman's health.)

There currently is no cure. Warts may be removed with caustic solutions, creams, freezing, burning, lasers, or surgery, but the external, visible warts are not the ones that put you at risk of cervical cancer. However, the dangerous types may be eliminated at the same time. Many women with condyloma first learn of them when they have an abnormal Pap smear since the virus is often present in tissue that shows precancerous changes.

Although condoms are better than no protection from condyloma, warts can occur in areas that aren't covered by a condom. Fortunately, condoms do protect well against the types of HPV that can inhabit the cervix.

Genital Herpes

Herpes is the most common STD in the United States. It infects nearly 22 percent of adults, or 40 million people. One reason that herpes incidence has expanded by 30 percent since 1983 is that more than half the carriers don't know they have it. For many people the initial symptoms of herpes are mild. (A blood test is available, but it's not reliable.) The herpes recurs later and may be more obvious then. An outbreak of herpes causes groups of painful small bumps on the genitals or other sensitive areas about twelve days (but sometimes much longer) after exposure to the virus. The person also feels as if he or she has the flu. If the person touches the sores, he or she can infect other parts of the body. Herpes can be fatal to a newborn.

Herpes is passed only by contact with the skin of an infected person. Although it's most contagious when sores are present, about 80 percent of transmissions take place when there are no symptoms. There are two types of herpes: I and II. Most Type II occurs below the waist, and most Type I above it.

There is no cure, but acyclovir (Zovirax), famciclovir (Famvir), and valacyclovir (Valtrex) reduce symptoms and will lessen recurrences if taken regularly. They may also reduce the likelihood of transmission, although there are not enough data yet to be sure. Condoms help reduce the risk of passing herpes to another person, but they still leave some areas uncovered.

When one partner has herpes, the couple faces a tough decision. Should they take protective measures into the foreseeable future and hope medicine will find a cure? Or should they assume it's inevitable that both will eventually be infected? (One study found that about 10 percent of couples in this situation get infected within a year despite using condoms.) It's not a simple choice, but it's one you should make together and not by default.

Gonorrhea

Once a top STD, gonorrhea receives a lot less attention in the AIDS era. As nearly 350,000 Americans found out in 1995, however, it's definitely still around. Gonorrhea is a bacterial infection that develops one to ten days after exposure and may present no symptoms at all, especially in women. In a man gonorrhea may cause burning on urination and a clear-to-cloudy discharge from the tip of the penis.

If gonorrhea isn't treated promptly, it may invade other parts of the urinary tract. A woman is at risk of developing pelvic inflammatory disease and tubal pregnancy. In men the urethra may narrow or sterility may result. Fortunately, most strains of gonorrhea respond to antibiotics.

Condoms are good insurance against the transmission of gonorrhea.

Hepatitis

Hepatitis is an inflammation of the liver that causes flu-like symptoms and occasionally jaundice, yellowed skin and eyes. Like HIV, hepatitis is caused by a virus, but some forms are nearly one hundred times as infectious from sexual contact. There are now seven types of hepatitis virus—A through G—and the list is likely to continue to grow. Only B and D are frequently transmitted through sexual contact, although Type A can be, and we don't know how half of Type C cases were transmitted.

Hepatitis B infection produces tiredness, muscle and joint pain, sore throat, fever, and gastrointestinal distress six weeks to six months after exposure. About 10 percent of cases become chronic and can cause liver disease. A vaccine is available for hepatitis B, and it's routinely given to children, health care workers, pregnant women, and others at risk.

Only people who have hepatitis B develop Type D. Intravenous drug use and sexual contact are the main modes of transmission. Type D may be either temporary or chronic, and is often more severe than type B alone. About 70 percent of those with hepatitis D develop cirrhosis of the liver.

None of the hepatitis viruses is easily treated once it's taken hold. That's why prevention—through safe sex or vaccination—is so important. Condoms are a key part of prevention, but bear in mind that hepatitis can be present in other bodily fluids besides blood, semen, and vaginal secretions.

Pubic Lice

Crab lice are tiny insects that take up residence in pubic hair and occasionally in hair on the head, beard, buttocks, thighs, or eyebrows. They walk there, usually during sexual contact. Condoms don't help prevent the spread. Lice may also reside in bedding for short periods, so it's important to clean bedding frequently if they're a problem. Crab lice produce itching and a rash about a month after exposure. Other difficulties are rare, although infections can develop. Crab lice are more a nuisance than a health problem. They can be eradicated by over-the-counter preparations.

Syphilis

Here's another old standard that doesn't get much publicity these days. As with gonorrhea, though, no news isn't necessarily good news. Rates hit a low in 1977 and have varied since then, with a recent high of 135,000 reported U.S. cases in 1990. Syphilis is contagious only when there are open sores— undoubtedly one reason that its reach is somewhat smaller than diseases that can be transmitted by people with no symptoms. The fact that it still continues shows that many people aren't using condoms, which are effective at preventing the spread.

Syphilis produces dull red spots on the skin ten to thirty days after exposure. The spots become pimples, eventually open and expand to form round or oval craters, and usually heal without ever causing any pain. A week to six months after the first episode, syphilis returns as a rash. Once the rash disappears, there may be no further symptoms until internal organs become infected and begin to deteriorate. Untreated, syphilis leads to dementia and death. Al Capone may have evaded the federal government and the mob, but he didn't practice safe sex. Syphilis killed him. Syphilis can be treated with antibiotics, ideally as soon as symptoms appear.

Trichomoniasis

Trichomoniasis, an infection by a protozoan (single-celled animal), is difficult to diagnose in men. Although about 70 percent of all men who have sex with an infected woman get it, only 5 to 10 percent develop symptoms (pain on urination and discharge), and some men get rid of the infection naturally within a few weeks. Women, however, develop a foul-smelling vaginal discharge that doesn't readily clear itself and may be passed off as a vaginal infection. If the infection is not treated, it can cause infertility. Fortunately, treatment with metronidazole is usually very effective. Condoms are helpful in preventing transmission.

Ureaplasma

Ureaplasma is diagnosed by ruling out other STDs. It has only been recognized in recent years as a disease distinct from gonorrhea. About 80 percent of women and 34 percent of men have no symptoms. Women may have a white discharge or lower abdominal pain.

Ureaplasma can lead to sterility, miscarriage, and premature birth in women, and epididymal and prostate problems in men. It may also cause rheumatic diseases such as infectious arthritis. Fortunately, antibiotics knock it out, and the spread can be prevented by using condoms.

Nonspecific Infections

This is a catchall classification for the remaining 10 percent of infections that may be linked to sexual activity, though we're not sure. For example, one particularly common problem among women, bacterial vaginitis, appears to be more prevalent in women with STDs, yet it doesn't seem to be spread by sexual contact. Men sometimes develop urethral infections that can't easily be diagnosed. Fortunately, most of these infections respond readily to antibiotics.

How to Use a Condom

When a woman meets resistance from a man over condoms, she may have to be the one responsible for supplying them and producing them at the right moment. Sure, guys ought to be taking charge of the one method of disease protection and temporary birth control that's male centered. In the real world, where not every man is as enlightened as we might like, it's vital for women to know how to protect themselves.

One option that gives the woman control is the female condom. Used properly it's as effective as the male condom at preventing disease and pregnancy. You insert it like a diaphragm. Like the diaphragm, practice makes perfect. It's better if you don't have to figure it out at the spur of the moment. For more about the female condom, see the following chapter, "Father Not to Be."

A woman can also supply and apply a male condom. Here's how to do it right:
• Only latex or polyurethane, non-novelty condoms protect against disease. Don't use condoms that are old or that have been stored in an adverse environment—a wallet, for example. Never use natural or exotic condoms for disease prevention. Natural condoms are a sufficient barrier to sperm but cannot block the much smaller organisms that cause disease. Lubrication with the spermicide nonoxynol-9 increases protection against some diseases, including HIV.

• The condom should be on the man's penis before there's any other contact that involves his penis.

• Leave a space for semen at the tip of the condom. This can be done by squeezing the tip between index finger and thumb, and then rolling the condom all the way to the base of the penis.

• Never use an oil-based lubricant such as petroleum jelly, mineral or vegetable oil, or cold cream with a condom. Water-based lubricants such as KY Jelly are okay.

What to Say if He Doesn't Want to Use a Condom

Guys have a limited repertoire of excuses for not using a condom, so it's easy for you to be ready with a gentle and positive response.

• **"Sex won't feel as good."** The first thing to say is that they don't bother you at all. In fact, you like condoms because sex lasts longer when he wears one. Besides, you both can relax and have a really good time if you don't have to worry about disease or pregnancy. It probably wouldn't hurt to mention that you enjoy putting them on.

• **"Condoms spoil the mood."** The way to outmaneuver this complaint is to make it untrue. Applying a condom can be just as much fun as any other part of lovemaking—in fact, it needs to be in order to become a regular part of your sexual relationship.

• **"I have great control and can withdraw in time."** You could say that withdrawal doesn't prevent pregnancy or disease. You'll be more successful, though, if you insist that you don't want him to have to concentrate on that; you'd rather he concentrate on you, and a condom will take his mind off the problem of timely withdrawal.

• **"I'm allergic to rubber."** Although it's not very common, some people are allergic to latex rubber. To circumvent this complaint, simply be sure you have a supply of polyurethane condoms on hand. No one has yet reported an allergy to them.

• **"If you loved me, you wouldn't ask me to."** This claim is so absurd that it's difficult to take seriously. Nonetheless, if it comes up, you need only explain that you use condoms because you *do* love him and want him to be protected from any possible harm.

• **"They don't fit right and aren't comfortable."** Condoms are sold in different sizes, so why not have a fitting party—like a trip to the tailor in your own bedroom? What man can resist having a big deal made of his penis?

- The man should withdraw his penis immediately after ejaculating (while it's still erect), holding the condom in place at the base of the penis so it doesn't slip.
- Never reuse a condom.
- Combinations of methods improve protection. A diaphragm, cervical cap, or sponge provides some protection against STDs (not nearly as much as a condom), so combine a female-based method with a condom for the best possible protection.

A Word to the Wise

Most married women imagine that their monogamous relationship relieves them from worrying about sexually transmitted diseases. It is true that short of abstinence, a long-term monogamous relationship is the best protection from STDs. Unfortunately, monogamy is more often actually serial monogamy— one relationship to the next. He may be faithful to you now, but did he have partners before you? And, to be frank, even good men and husbands have been known to slip. STDs definitely are most common among the young and single, but my files are littered with cases involving older men and, too often, older couples. Take my word for it: Being eighty is no protection.

Please don't live your life in perpetual distrust and fear. Trust is the basis of any relationship. But be realistic. Ignoring signs of philandering will only put both of you at risk. All it takes is one misstep.

Even if your life is secure from the threat of STDs, if you have children, you still have plenty to worry about. Teaching abstinence is useful, but it isn't enough. Young people need information, not just prohibitions. A study of ninth graders, reported in the *Journal of Pediatrics,* found that three factors predict risky sexually behavior: peer pressure, alcohol and drug use, and lack of knowledge about sexually transmitted diseases. By instruction and example we should teach our children to resist the first two risk factors, but we can only be certain of success with the third. Frank talk is the solution.

The days of popping a pill to erase the effects of a one-night stand are long gone. Too many STDs, and especially the most dangerous ones, become permanent problems. They can ruin relationships and lives. Do what you can to keep your loved ones safe from their threat. Don't forget to protect yourself, too.

17

Father-*Not*-to-Be

Children are the ultimate blessing for many of us, but their arrival is usually more welcome at certain times of our lives than others. If you trust the timing to your lucky stars, you'll probably get an unpleasant surprise. If you and your partner have unprotected intercourse every other day, the odds are one in three that you'll be pregnant by the end of the month. If you have sex once a week, your odds are 15 percent, giving you six months to a year before you get pregnant. Each year at least half of all pregnancies in the United States are unintended, resulting in more than one million abortions and 2 million unplanned births.

Most couples prefer to control their childbearing with contraception, otherwise known as birth control or family planning. Contraception should be a joint responsibility, but there's a strong possibility you'll have to take care of the details. There are far more female than male forms of birth control. I wish I could tell you a revolution in male birth control is right around the corner, but it'll probably be five years before anything new reaches the market.

However, birth control should not be your responsibility alone. Your partner should be as informed as you are about the relative merits and demerits of the various approaches, he should participate in decisions about methods, and, to whatever degree possible, he should be involved in implementing them. There are no decisions you'll make as a couple that are as important as deciding whether to have children and how to control the timing.

Remember that many methods of birth control offer absolutely no protection against disease. Methods that do protect from disease may not be the best ways for you to prevent pregnancy. Be clear about what you're trying to accomplish. Male and female condoms, supplemented by spermicides, are the only good choices if your most important goal is preventing disease. In this chapter we'll be talking only about pregnancy prevention.

Each method of birth control has pros and cons. Base your choice on who you are and where you are in life. If you and your relationship are young, and you either plan to have children later or want to leave the possibility open, you're looking for temporary contraception. If you're certain you don't want children or that your childbearing years are behind you, you're in the market for permanent birth control.

By the way, not everyone does want children, and there's nothing wrong

---

Does It Work?

Effectiveness will probably be your first question about any method of birth control. Here are statistics from the Allen Guttmacher Institute, a leader in research about reproduction. Some methods are more effective than others. Note that even a very effective method fails sometimes; if a technique is 97 percent effective, three out of one hundred couples who use it will have a pregnancy *each year*. The chart shows both "perfect use" and "average use." When you compare the two, you'll see that some methods are more likely than others to fail because they aren't used properly. For example, although the pill can be more effective than an IUD, it fails more often because the woman must remember to take it.

This chart shows estimates of the percentage of women who have an unintended pregnancy in the first year of using a method.

METHOD	PERFECT USE	AVERAGE USE
None (chance)	85	85
Spermicides	3	30
Sponge	8	24
Withdrawal	4	24
Periodic abstinence	9	19
Cervical cap	6	18
Diaphragm	6	18
Condom	2	16
Pill	0.1	6
IUD	0.8	4
Tubal ligation	0.2	0.5
Depo-Provera	0.3	0.4
Vasectomy	0.1	0.2
Norplant	0.04	0.05

with that. I once knew a surgeon who used to bang his fist on his desk and say that he wouldn't perform a vasectomy on a man unless he had two children, had been married at least ten years, and was older than thirty-five. Who ordained him? That's an inappropriate attitude for a medical professional. As long as a couple approaches permanent birth control responsibly and is aware of the options, it's their decision.

Now I'll step down from my soapbox and discuss the methods. Let's talk about the temporary methods first, then permanent ones. The following discussion will be general, with a focus on the ways a man can participate. For more information about female-based methods, talk with your gynecologist.

Temporary Male Contraceptives

Male Condom

The most basic barrier method, the male condom is very effective when used properly. The more dedicated you and your partner are to proper use, the better you can expect condoms to work for you. Condoms are also the only form of birth control that offer some protection from STDs. In addition they're simple to use, economical, and without side effects. (Some people are allergic to latex, but there are also condoms made from polyurethane and from animals. Both prevent pregnancy, but the animal-based condoms offer no disease protection.)

Condoms do require a pause in foreplay, but an inventive couple can turn that into fun. Some men (and few women) think they interfere with sensation, but for a man prone to ejaculate before he would like to, that can be a benefit. (Condoms are not a solution for real premature ejaculation; see chapter 15.) It can be a bother that the man's penis must be removed from the woman's vagina immediately after ejaculation.

For information on how to choose and use condoms, see chapter 16.

Withdrawal

This method is free, always available, and better than nothing at all. Effectiveness? Well, there's a greater range than for any other method. For the man with perfect control who ejaculates well away from the woman's vulva, the rate might go as high as 96 percent. (Almost all penises emit some pre-ejaculate that can contain sperm.) In actual practice, however, effectiveness is more like 76 percent—better than going for broke, but the odds are going to catch up with you before long.

Nonpenetrative Sex

If sperm can't reach the egg, there will be no pregnancy, so preventing sperm from getting in or near the vagina is 100 percent effective birth control. (Of course, so is abstinence.) "Outercourse," as it has been called, can be fun and satisfying, but for how long? For couples who prefer not to use "artificial" birth control solutions (for religious or other reasons), nonpenetrative sex—manual or oral stimulation for mutual satisfaction—may be effectively combined with periodic abstinence.

On the Horizon

Frankly, there's not a great deal of research into any form of birth control, let alone male-based forms. Pharmaceutical companies are leery of legal pitfalls, and government agencies have been reluctant to move into such a politically sensitive area. There has been some promising work, though.

Most men who are injected with a form of testosterone (and sometimes progestin) every twelve weeks cease to produce sperm. (All of them have at least a marked reduction.) Sex drive remains the same, and fertility returns not long after the injections are stopped. This approach was tested first in Europe and has only recently begun trials in the United States, where its effectiveness has been in the high 90 percent range. If continuing trials show that this method is both effective and safe, it could be available as early as 2001.

Other scientists are developing chemicals which inhibit the enzymes that help sperm locate and bind to eggs. In effect these drugs make sperm blind. Developed at North Carolina State University, this approach has been tested on laboratory rats and found more than 90 percent effective. Investigators hope to start human trials of an oral contraceptive in about five years.

Temporary Female Contraceptives

Female Condom

The female condom is a relative newcomer. Its advantages are that it's under the woman's control, it's made of polyurethane (nonallergenic), it can be put in place in advance of sex, and it remains effective if the man's penis isn't erect. The difference in effectiveness between "perfect use" and "average use" is greater for the female than for the male condom. Although female condoms may be a good choice for occasional use, they may not be a good choice for regular contraception because many people seem to have trouble using them properly.

Diaphragm and Cervical Cap

Both the diaphragm and cervical cap block sperm's passage into the cervix. The diaphragm is larger and covers the end of the vagina, and the cap covers the cervix alone. Both are available by prescription and cost less than $25 (plus the doctor's visit). Effectiveness is typically about 82 percent for either, although the cervical cap doesn't work well if the woman has had a child (effectiveness drops as low as 55 percent). Either device can be inserted before intercourse (no more than two hours before for the diaphragm, and no less than twenty minutes before for the cap), and both must be left in place for six hours after intercourse. The diaphragm may be left in place as long as eight hours, the cap forty-eight. Placement should be checked and more spermicide applied before subsequent intercourse.

Side effects of diaphragms and caps are both positive and negative. A regular diaphragm user may experience more bladder infections, but her risk of cervical dysplasia and cancer is slightly less. Both devices may reduce the risk of pelvic inflammatory disease. Because of the spermicidal jelly, the methods are a bit messy (the cap less so because it's smaller).

Intrauterine Device (IUD)

An IUD is a device inserted by a doctor through the vagina into the uterus, where it appears to change cervical mucus in a way that prevents sperm from reaching a fallopian tube. As you can see on the chart, the IUD does this very effectively.

IUDs are more widely used outside the United States than in it. Worldwide the IUD is the most common form of temporary contraception. As recently as 1982, about 7 percent of U.S. women chose it as their contraceptive, but by 1990 that number had declined to 1 percent. The reason can be summed up in two words: Dalkon Shield. In the 1980s that brand of IUD, and that brand only, was associated with a risk of infection. Continuing experience has shown that IUDs are a safe form of birth control for many women. They are recognized as such by the World Health Organization, the American Medical Association, and the American College of Obstetricians.

A doctor must insert (or remove) an IUD, so although the device isn't expensive in itself, it may cost a few hundred dollars to have one inserted. The device typically can stay in place for eight to ten years. (Models with the hormone progesterone must be replaced annually.)

Few gynecologists recommend IUDs for women who haven't had at least one child because the risk of expulsion is greater. Most expulsions occur in the first three months. The most common side effects are increased bleeding and cramping during periods. There is a very small chance (one to three in one thousand) the uterus will be punctured during insertion. Also, when an IUD fails, the pregnancy is more likely than usual to be ectopic (in the fallopian tubes), which can be very dangerous.

One reason the IUD is so effective is that it does its job without requiring that the man or woman do anything. The only maintenance required is to check after each period to make sure the plastic string that extends through the cervix a short distance into the vagina is present and no longer than usual. This shows the IUD is still in place. Your partner could learn to perform that task.

Spermicides

By themselves, spermicides aren't effective contraceptives, but they boost the effectiveness of barrier methods like the diaphragm and condom. Spermicides are available as creams, gels, foams, suppositories, and a film that is placed against the cervix. Nearly all contain nonoxynol-9. The film is effective for about two hours, the rest only one. All can be messy. Spermicides may be female centered, but they certainly can be a cooperative venture.

The Pill

The combination birth control pill, containing the two main female hormones, estrogen and progestin (synthetic progesterone), prevents pregnancy by interfering with the natural cycle of hormones and by thickening the cervical mucus, which bars sperm from the uterus. The pill has changed a lot since its early days. The doses are much smaller, reducing side effects, and are sometimes varied during the menstrual cycle. A study at San Francisco State University found that pills which provide three different doses during the menstrual cycle (triphasic pills) may enhance a woman's sexual interest and response. All forms of combination birth control pills are highly effective—as long as you remember to take them.

Many women experience no side effects from the pill, and those who do usually have minor problems and for only the first few cycles: spotting between periods, nausea, breast enlargement and tenderness, headaches, and fluid retention. If these problems persist, a different pill may help. Women who are breast-feeding a baby should not take the pill.

Most long-term health effects are positive, providing the woman doesn't smoke. (Smokers over age thirty-five shouldn't take the pill because of increased risk of heart attack and stroke.) Women who take the pill enjoy some protection from ovarian and endrometrial cancer, pelvic inflammatory disease, osteoporosis, and breast lumps. The pill does not increase the risk of breast cancer.

Minipill

The minipill contains only progestin. It can be a good choice for women who have continuing side effects with the pill, who shouldn't take the pill because of health problems (such as smoking), or who are breast-feeding a baby. The minipill is nearly as effective as the pill, but there is less margin for error. It has to be taken every day at about the same time. Because the minipill is taken every day, it blocks ovulation and regular periods, although the woman may bleed at irregular intervals.

Implants

Pellets about 1½ inches long are inserted under the skin of the inside upper arm. They release a steady supply of progestin into the bloodstream, preventing ovulation and thickening cervical mucus. The implants last about five years, when they can be replaced, and are even more effective than the pill (because you don't have to remember to take them). Most healthy women experience few side effects, the most common being irregular bleeding. Nonetheless, it's a good idea to test your reaction to progestin-based contraceptives first, since the implants are more difficult to discontinue than a pill or shot.

Injections

Another way to deliver progestin is by injection every three months. Like other forms of progestin-based birth control, injections can cause irregular bleeding. After a year or so, however, most women cease having periods altogether. Like implants, injections can cause weight gain or mood changes. For women with epilepsy, injections can be a good choice since they decrease the frequency of seizures.

Emergency Contraception

The so-called morning-after pill can actually be taken up to seventy-two hours after intercourse, although its effectiveness drops over that period.

There are several different hormonal approaches used worldwide, and it's not entirely clear how they work. The pill used most often in the United States contains a combination of estrogen and progestin, and seems to inhibit ovulation. The effectiveness of morning-after pills seems to be between about 75 percent and nearly 100 percent, depending on when in the woman's cycle it is administered.

Emergency contraception should be just that. It's appropriate only when something goes wrong—for example, a condom tears. Nonetheless, it's important to know that there is help when the unexpected happens.

Planned Abstinence

The success of planned abstinence, sometimes called natural family planning, depends on your awareness of your menstrual cycle and the biology of reproduction. Using a variety of techniques—the calendar, body temperature, and cervical mucus—you attempt to estimate when you ovulate and avoid unprotected intercourse for seven days before and three days after. Because sperm can live in the fallopian tubes up to seven days and the egg survives up to twenty-four hours after ovulation, this approach prevents the two from taking up residence together.

Planned abstinence requires a significant amount of observation and record keeping, and a willingness of both the man and woman to forgo unprotected intercourse for ten days per month—or up to half the time between periods. On the plus side, both partners can help and will learn a great deal about the reproductive cycle. The results, depending on how carefully it's practiced, can be good.

Permanent Birth Control

The female surgical procedure called tubal ligation is the most widely practiced form of birth control in the United States. It has been chosen by nearly 30 percent of all users of contraception, and its popularity continues to grow despite the fact that vasectomy, the male alternative, is easier, more effective, less dangerous, and less costly. Nonetheless, tubal ligation is a very effective way to end your childbearing years, so let's look into it.

As the name suggests, tubal ligation closes off the fallopian tubes so that eggs can no longer pass. The surgery usually costs between $1,000 and $2,500, somewhat less if done at the same time as a cesarean section. Although it can be done with a small incision (laparoscopically) and as an outpatient, it still usually requires general anesthetic, which carries some inherent risks. Possible complications are the same as for any surgical procedure: a small chance of infection, bleeding, or damage to adjacent organs. The failure rate for tubal ligation is very low, but when it does fail, tubal pregnancy, which can be life-threatening, is much more likely. The complications and success of the surgery depend on the skill of the surgeon, so choose carefully.

The male version of permanent birth control is the vasectomy. To my way of thinking, vasectomy is the logical choice for couples who are certain they want no (or no more) children. The simple procedure can be performed in a doctor's office under local anesthetic and completed in fifteen minutes or less. It usually costs between $350 and $500. Because the vasa deferentia are near the surface of the scrotum, it's easy to access them, cut them, and seal their ends. In fact, many urologists, myself included, now use a technique and tool developed by the Chinese called "no-scalpel" vasectomy. Without an incision the tool is used to grasp the vas deferens, make a tiny puncture, and retrieve it for closure. No stitches are required, and there's generally little discomfort. As long as the man spends the next forty-eight hours off his feet and applies ice packs, pain medicine usually isn't needed. A few men react to the local anesthetic; occasionally there is bleeding (more likely with a standard vasectomy); infection occurs in about 4 percent of men with a standard vasectomy; sperm granulomas (lumps caused by the immune system attacking leaked sperm) form and cause problems in about 2 percent of cases; testicles may ache, but this usually disappears within six months; or the epididymis might become inflamed, which usually clears up within a week. Each of these complications is rare, is generally less severe than a complication from tubal ligation, and, unlike tubal ligation, no one has ever died from a vasectomy.

Men's discomfort over the idea of some other man handling that area of their body—with a knife in hand!—has produced a lot of creative fiction about vasectomies. Men pass around lots of horror stories about swelling and pain. I think one of the most common fears, though, is the shot of anesthetic. A lot of guys ask whether I will really be putting a shot into their testes. In fact, it goes into the skin, and most guys say it hurts more to get a shot of Novocain at the dentist. Men also occasionally perpetuate myths about the vasectomy's effect on the quality of sex. In truth, it has no effect on erections or the experience of ejaculation, and it does not alter sex drive at all. Indeed, many men report an increase in libido, probably because the worry of pregnancy is gone.

Vasectomy is very effective, but in about 0.1 percent of cases the vasa deferentia grow back together again. This can happen at any time but becomes less likely as time goes by. More often the method fails because couples fail to heed warnings that sperm may remain in the man's reproductive tract for quite some time after the procedure. As a general rule it takes at least twenty ejaculations to remove all living sperm. Protection should be used until a semen test shows that sperm are absent.

The long-term health effects of a vasectomy have been extensively studied, and nothing serious has been found. There used to be some concern about an association with prostate cancer, but intense analysis, including a panel of the National Institutes of Health, found little or no association, although the panel did recommend further research, none of which has shown an increased risk of prostate cancer in men who have had vasectomies. About two-thirds of men who have had a vasectomy have sperm antibodies in their blood. This doesn't appear to cause any problems unless a man hopes for vasectomy reversal.

A few men develop psychological or sexual problems because they've rushed into a vasectomy. The choice of vasectomy should be thoroughly discussed

---

Considering a Vasectomy

These are signs that vasectomy would be a good choice:
- You both have all the children you ever want to have.
- You have a stable, long-term relationship.
- You can't or don't want to use temporary methods.
- One of you has a medical condition that precludes other methods.
- You have a condition that makes pregnancy risky.
- You want to enjoy intercourse without fear of pregnancy.

These are signs that vasectomy might *not* be the right choice:
- Either of you is young.
- You have no or few children.
- Your relationship is unstable.
- Either of you feels pressure from the other to have a vasectomy.
- You don't want him to have a vasectomy, but he's pushing for it.
- Either of you might want to have children in the future.
- Either of you thinks it might solve an emotional, marital, or sexual problem.
- Your partner has a condition that makes elective surgery risky.
- Either of you imagines that vasectomy is reversible.

---

beforehand, and both partners should agree. Any hint of concern should make you both wary.

About two of one thousand men who have vasectomies eventually end up regretting the decision and try for reversal. Most often they do so because their life circumstances have changed and they want another child, not because of psychological distress. I'll discuss reversal in the next chapter, but I want to emphasize that it's expensive, difficult, and far from sure. When choosing a vasectomy, every man should consider it permanent.

Because vasectomy is in my area of medical expertise, I've gone to some length to fully inform you about it, including the rare complications. I want to assure you that I've seen the positives far more often than the negatives. For couples that are ready for it, vasectomy may be the ideal form of permanent birth control. Most couples feel great relief to be freed from worries of pregnancy. About 30 percent report that they have more sex and enjoy it more after a vasectomy. At least 90 percent of men would do it again and would recommend it to friends. More than 95 percent of women whose partners have a vasectomy report satisfaction with the procedure.

Sharing the Decisions

For too many women, birth control is a lonely business. They make the choices and take care of business on their own, simply out of self-preservation. It shouldn't and doesn't have to be so. Many men have thought of birth control as the woman's responsibility simply because most forms are woman-based. It's time they joined the partnership and took responsibility for your joint fertility.

As a first step, discuss the contraceptive choices with him. If the method you're using now isn't ideal, talk over the other options and ask for his opinion. For that matter there's nothing wrong with suggesting that he take charge occasionally and bring along a condom. Most men aren't opposed to taking part; they just don't know the ropes. Help him learn them, and you'll be a happier couple.

18

Father-to-Be

Your career is established, you've traded in the roadster for a minivan, you have a spare bedroom, and your gynecologist has cleared you for conception. It's time to start a family.

You studied your role, but what is your partner's? Beyond their obvious initial contribution and handing out cigars, many men don't know what's involved in fatherhood. Let me help. I'll line up plenty for him to do, from well before conception to past the arrival. First, let's look at what he should and shouldn't do to increase the likelihood of conception and a healthy fetus.

Behaving Like a Father-to-Be

Until a few years ago doctors thought that a man either had viable sperm or he didn't, and that those sperm either carried genetic abnormalities or they didn't. Boy, were we wrong. Although studies are just being undertaken, we're already alarmed by how much a man's health and his environment can affect sperm. How your partner behaves when you're trying to conceive may make a big difference.

For example, smoking profoundly influences semen and the sperm it contains. A variety of studies since 1990 have shown that tobacco smoke can reduce ejaculate volume, sperm density, and sperm motility (their activity), and increase the proportion of abnormally shaped sperm. These can all reduce a man's fertility. There are other concerns as well. A five-year study of in vitro fertilization patients at the State University of New York at Stony Brook showed a nearly 65 percent increase in miscarriages when the father or both partners smoked. We also know that children of male smokers have an increased risk of leukemia. We don't know whether the abnormal sperm or some other factor increased the miscarriages or leukemia, but these findings are more reasons for him to give up cigarettes.

Heavy drinking also reduces male fertility. It appears that the alcohol reduces both testosterone and sperm production, although the exact mechanism isn't yet clear. Moderate drinking doesn't cause such problems, but caution is in order here as well since we don't know much about how alcohol might affect the health of the sperm produced.

Marijuana's influence on sperm quality has been quite controversial, as has just about everything associated with cannabis. Smoking the weed clearly reduces sperm density and motility, and increases the number of abnormal sperm, just as tobacco smoke does. How it does so, however, is less clear. Some research has shown a decrease in the levels of male hormones in marijuana smokers; other research has not. Whatever the cause, the damage to sperm is clear. Why take chances?

How serious is he about his physique? He wouldn't consider taking steroids, would he? Anabolic steroids suppress sperm production and motility, and reduce the percentage of normal sperm. In most cases, quitting steroids returns normal sperm production, but some cases of ongoing infertility have been recorded.

Other behaviors that may help and can't hurt include keeping caffeine to a minimum (no more than two cups of coffee per day), avoiding situations that keep his testes too warm (no hot tubs, saunas, or tight underwear), and taking a multivitamin that includes vitamin C.

In sum, for the best chance of a quick conception and a healthy baby, your partner ought to do all those things that would preserve and improve his health anyway. Besides avoiding the toxins mentioned above, he should eat well and get regular exercise. Neither is known to have any direct effect on sperm quality, but being overweight can dampen ardor, and exercise does seem to help maintain youthful testosterone levels and increase interest in sex.

Threats to Male Fertility

Despite the best behavior, many men do have trouble conceiving a baby. Between 20 and 35 percent of couples fail to achieve pregnancy after a year of trying, and the root of the problem is about equally on the male and female sides. Since this book is about men for women, I'll discuss only the male side of the equation here. But when conception proves difficult, both the man and woman should be checked by a doctor—a urologist in his case and an obstetrician/gynecologist in hers.

When you and your partner have a fertility problem that proves to be male based, you should expect a significant psychological reaction from him. In most men's minds, fertility is intimately tied to virility—and therefore to manhood. It can be a first-order threat to his image of himself as a man. Depression is common among men with infertility, although anger and even disbelief aren't unusual. One of my patients' reaction to the news that he had nearly a zero sperm count was so severe that it eventually broke their marriage apart. I encouraged him to talk to a counselor about it, but he refused. His attitude and behavior went steadily downhill until his wife couldn't stand it any longer.

Unfortunately, the incidence of infertility has increased in the past thirty-five years, and there is evidence, though controversial, that one reason is an overall decline in sperm count in men in industrialized countries. The ways in which a man's fertility can be compromised are numerous, but they can be divided into two general categories: testicular and chemical.

Problems with the Testes

There are numerous physical problems in the testes that can cause infertility.

One is a history of undescended testicles. Normally while a male fetus is developing in the uterus, his testes descend from near the kidneys into the scrotum. Less than 1 percent of the time, the testes still haven't descended by the first birthday. If the condition is not treated, it will cause permanent infertility. Some damage may occur by as early as the end of the second year. Parents of a boy with cryptorchidism (the medical term for the condition) should have the problem corrected promptly and should let him know later in his life that he had it.

If a testicle (rarely both testes) becomes twisted, called testicular torsion, its blood supply can be cut off; if the situation continues for long, the testicle will be damaged. Testicular torsion is unusual among older men, but it happens to one in four thousand males younger than twenty-five. It requires immediate medical attention. Sometimes the testicle can be untwisted, but surgery is often required to prevent infertility.

An impact to the testes can reduce fertility, although this seems to be relatively rare. Still, boys and men should wear athletic protectors when playing sports.

Varicocele, enlargement of the veins in the spermatic cord, is one of the most common causes of male infertility (one estimate is as high as 41 percent). Varicoceles often start in early puberty (about 15 percent of thirteen-year-olds have them) and progress with age. They can cause the testes to atrophy and produce less testosterone. Unfortunately, there are few symptoms of a varicocele, and few men know anything about them. An advanced varicocele resembles a mass of worms in the scrotum just above the testes. Most of the time only the left side is affected, but occasionally both sides are. To detect a varicocele at an earlier stage, your partner should take a warm shower to relax his scrotum. After he gets out, and while he's still warm and standing, he should flex his pelvic muscles as if he's trying to have a bowel movement. As he does this, look for bulging, bluish veins. Then he should lie down and relax; look to see if the veins have collapsed. Varicoceles can readily be treated by a urologist. An outpatient technique called varicocelectomy has the best chance of success and the fewest complications. This technique restores fertility between 50 and 70 percent of the time. Still, the earlier the problem is detected, the better the chance of success.

Infections can also harm the testes. Among adult men who get mumps, a third have inflamed testes (orchitis), which leads to infertility 87 percent of the time. Nearly all young males in the United States have been vaccinated against mumps. Several sexually transmitted diseases can scar or block the ejaculatory duct, vasa deferentia, or epididymis. Chlamydia, gonorrhea, and ureaplasma can lead to male (and female) infertility.

Problems with Medications and Toxins

We've already talked about the effects of smoking, drinking, and marijuana on fertility. Some prescription medications and chemical toxins can cause infertility, too. In most cases these changes are permanent, although sperm counts improve later in some cases.

Among medications, certain antibiotics are probably the most common culprits. Tetracyclines and erythromycin, for example, can affect sperm motility. If you're having trouble conceiving and your partner is taking antibiotics, he definitely should talk with his doctor about switching to a different antibiotic. Other drugs that can reduce fertility are the blood pressure medications called calcium-channel blockers and some drugs for inflammatory bowel disease, ulcers, and gout.

Your partner's fertility could also be affected if his own mother took diethylstilbestrol (DES), during her pregnancy. This is related to the much more widely known health problems of daughters whose mothers took DES, including increased risk of vaginal and cervical cancer. During the evaluation that we'll discuss later, the doctor should ask your husband if his mother took DES, so he ought to find out.

Occupational exposure to certain chemicals reduces or eliminates male fertility. For example, the pesticide dibromochloropropane (DBCP) was widely used until it was discovered that it lowered sperm counts. As many as 25 percent of banana workers have been diagnosed as infertile as a result of exposure. The replacement for DBCP are undoubtedly safer, but because we still know relatively little about how chemicals interact with male fertility, it's wise to limit exposure whenever possible. Men who work with lead have also been found to have low sperm counts, loss of sperm motility, and an unusual number of malformed sperm. Protective clothing and equipment help, but lead is eliminated from the body only slowly.

The extent of damage caused by man-made chemicals in the environment is poorly understood. As mentioned earlier, some research suggests that sperm counts in industrialized nations have been declining for several decades, and pollution has been implicated.

Maximizing the Likelihood of Conception

It's not unusual for couples to have trouble conceiving simply because they don't fully understand the biology of reproduction. One study of men examined for infertility found that 21 percent didn't know when their partner was most fertile. Timing makes a difference.

The window of opportunity for conception is about seven days, but the odds are best if you have intercourse within forty-eight hours of ovulation. It can help to predict ovulation through basal temperature and cervical mucus (see the section on natural family planning in the last chapter) or with a urine-test kit, but simply having intercourse every two days is nearly as good. Sperm can live in mucus for about two days, while the egg survives only twelve to twenty-four hours. As long as you keep sperm hanging around by regularly recharging the supply, the likelihood of pregnancy is good.

Why not have intercourse more often than every other day? Ejaculating more frequently than every forty-eight hours (no masturbation either!) may not allow his system to fully recharge the "sperm banks." (Waiting longer than five days is counterproductive because the sperm become less energetic.) Occasionally, it may help to break the two-day rule. If you're pretty sure you've timed ovulation accurately, have intercourse again as soon as he's ready. We now know that one ejaculation doesn't completely deplete the supply; the second one is sometimes quite rich in sperm.

It's a myth that women can't become pregnant unless they have an orgasm. Plenty of nonorgasmic women have become pregnant. Still, orgasm may help transport the sperm through the cervix. Also, the level of stimulation he achieves before ejaculation can make a difference. The more excited he becomes, the more semen—and therefore sperm—there will be. (That's why semen samples achieved by masturbation may not show a man's true sperm count.)

If you use a lubricant for intercourse, including oral sex as foreplay, it could well get in the way of conception. Saliva, KY Jelly, Lubifax, Surgilube, Keri Lotion, and most other commonly used sexual lubricants decrease sperm motility. Try olive oil instead.

The final technique that's likely to help is simply to lighten up a bit. Sex is supposed to be fun, but for too many couples who have trouble conceiving, it becomes a job. I've seen a number of men who became impotent because they felt pressure to perform on demand. Fortunately, they're among the easiest infertility patients to treat. All they need is a change in attitude.

If you're trying to get pregnant now, don't become too concerned by all the things that can go wrong. Only about 15 percent of couples fail to conceive by normal methods, and there are still plenty of options left to them. The odds are in your favor of raising a happy, healthy family—especially if you work together to take good care of each other, start at a relatively young age, and relax and enjoy it. Remember, this is supposed to be fun, not work.

Medicine to the Rescue

When the simpler measures don't work, medical science has an impressive array of more advanced techniques to offer the infertile male. Before any further steps are taken, he should see a urologist for a physical exam and a semen analysis. To be successful and economical, the treatment must be tailored to the problem rather than just attacked with high technology. Start with the basics and move on to specialists if it proves necessary.

Evaluation

After discussing the history of the problem—during which many of the factors mentioned above should come up—the urologist will do a physical exam. Obviously, the exam concentrates on the genitals, but it should include a check for secondary male characteristics, such as pubic hair, beard, and body build; this portion will be done with him standing up. The urologist will check his penis for curvature and for the location of the urethral opening, which could affect proper placement of semen in your vagina. Next comes a check of the testes for size and consistency; unusually small testes are often a sign of inadequate sperm production. A wide discrepancy in size suggests a varicocele, since varicoceles usually affect only the left side. The doctor will also feel for cysts or other abnormalities on the epididymis, the vasa deferentia, and the spermatic cord. Once again the greatest concern here is a varicocele. (Ultrasound can confirm the presence of a varicocele or even detect those too small to be felt, but this generally isn't necessary.)

A thorough semen analysis, a key part of an infertility examination, is considerably more than a sperm count. Even a standard test includes semen volume, sperm motility (movement), their forward progress, the percentage of abnormal sperm, a check for excess semen viscosity or clumping, and the presence of pus (showing infection). The accompanying table lists minimum values developed by my colleague Larry Lipshultz, a professor of medicine at Baylor College of Medicine. As Dr. Lipshultz would say, however, it's very difficult to define what normal is, and some men whose numbers are below these minimums may still be fertile.

Semen Test Results: Minimum Levels for Fertility	
Ejaculate volume	1.5–5.0 milliliters
Sperm density	greater than 20 million per milliliter
Motility	greater than 60 percent
Forward progression	greater than 2 (on a scale of 0 to 4)
Normal-shaped sperm	greater than 60 percent

In some cases none of the standard semen tests explains the cause of male infertility, and more complicated (and expensive) testing may be in order. Motility can be assessed with computer-based photography; the presence of pus can be analyzed using a semen culture or in great detail using monoclonal antibodies; an immunobead test can check for sperm antibodies produced by the immune system; the interaction of sperm and cervical mucus can be checked after intercourse; and a number of tests can check the ability of sperm to fertilize.

Although this may seem a bit odd, an infertility examination generally includes a urine test. An infertile man may be partially or totally ejaculating into his bladder rather than through his penis. The cause can be surgery, infection and scarring, or neurological problems (for example, diabetic neuropathy).

Finally, if sperm counts are very low or zero, the hormone levels in his blood will be tested. Abnormal hormone levels suggest a testicular problem. Normal hormone levels but no sperm often indicate an obstruction somewhere in the six meters of the man's sperm-delivery system.

Treatments for Male Infertility

Infertility treatment depends, of course, on the cause of the infertility. **Varicoceles** can be corrected with surgery, and semen quality usually improves. Infections can be treated with antibiotics.

A low volume of semen usually means that the ejaculatory duct in the prostate is obstructed or that the man is ejaculating partially or totally (retrograde ejaculation) into his bladder. In the former case, **obstruction** can be seen in an ultrasound image, and the ejaculatory duct can be opened up by surgery through the penis. **Retrograde ejaculation** can sometimes be treated with medications; in other cases the sperm can be collected from the urine and used for an assisted reproductive technology, such as in vitro fertilization.

Because sperm make up such a small part of the ejaculate (about 5 percent), semen volume doesn't tell much about potential blockages of the vasa deferentia or epididymis. Any blockages can be revealed by vasography, in which dye is injected to produce an X-ray image. Some such blockages can be corrected surgically; others may require aspiration of sperm from either the epididymis or the testes for use in an assisted reproductive technology.

If the problem is **low hormone levels,** the man can take supplemental hormones. However, abnormally high levels of some hormones called gonadotropins can also cause problems. A number of different medications have been used to treat such conditions, but their effectiveness is still controversial. In particular cases a testicular biopsy might be in order to rule out tumors or congenital conditions.

Assisted Reproductive Technologies

Although in vitro fertilization (IVF)—in which an egg and sperm are combined in the laboratory to produce a so-called test-tube baby—is the best-known technique for assisted reproduction, it is only one of more than a half-dozen approaches ranging from simple and inexpensive to complex and costly. Few insurance companies will cover the cost of assisted reproductive technologies, although some states now require it.

The simplest technique is called intrauterine insemination (IUI), or artificial insemination. At the time of ovulation, sperm are collected from the man by masturbation or a sperm-collection condom and washed to concentrate the normally shaped, active sperm. Then they are placed high in the woman's uterus using a catheter. Success is most likely when the man's semen quality is relatively good (my gynecologist friends say a sperm count of at least ten million) but a postintercourse test has indicated a problem at the cervix, such as a mucus incompatibility. In such cases the technique works between 15 and 20 percent of the time in each cycle; after six unsuccessful attempts, there's little point in continuing. Each attempt costs a few hundred dollars.

There are several forms of in vitro fertilization. The classic version involves stimulating the woman's ovaries by drug therapy, retrieving as many eggs as possible, mixing them with washed sperm, incubating the mixture for twenty-four to forty-eight hours, and placing some or all of the fertilized eggs (embryos) back in the uterus. (Unused embryos can be frozen for later attempts.) One variation on IVF eliminates the stimulation of the ovaries with drugs and is called natural-cycle IVF. Zygote intrafallopian transfer starts out the same as IVF, but the embryo is placed in a fallopian tube rather than in the uterus. In vitro fertilization may help when the semen has marginal quality but probably not poor quality. About 15 percent of couples become parents with IVF when male-factor infertility is involved. Each attempt may cost a few thousand dollars.

The first steps of gamete intrafallopian transfer (GIFT) are the same as in IVF, but the eggs and sperm aren't incubated in the laboratory. Instead they are mixed and placed in a fallopian tube where fertilization can take place in

The Psychological Stress of Infertility

The pursuit of fertility can be very stressful. If you choose to avail yourselves of everything that modern medicine has to offer, you can spend years—and tens of thousands of dollars—pursuing pregnancy. Consider the fact that you'll spend most of that time waiting in a state of high anxiety and that the news is more likely to be bad than good. Far too many couples don't really grasp the likelihood of success. For the unlucky, it's one disappointment after another.

Be very sure that both of you are truly behind any decisions you make about treatments. If the efforts to achieve pregnancy pull you apart rather than bring you together, stop, talk, and be sure you're doing the right thing.

the woman's body. Success rates for male-factor infertility with GIFT may approach 25 percent.

When semen quality is very low, micromanipulation techniques may be in order. If a few healthy, normal sperm are present in the ejaculate, one may be inserted into an egg to cause fertilization. When no sperm are present in the ejaculate, it may be possible to extract some from the epididymis or testes. The embryo can then be placed in the uterus or a fallopian tube. There are three degrees of invasiveness of the egg during micromanipulation, but the best success appears to be with intracytoplasmic sperm injection (ICSI). Success rates for ICSI approach 30 percent in some studies, at a cost of $7,000 to $12,000 per attempt.

Reversing a Vasectomy

A man who thought he wanted no more children can—because of the loss of a child or remarriage—find himself wishing for more. Although I tell my patients who are considering a vasectomy to think of it as permanent, it can often be reversed.

The chance of success depends on the length of time since the vasectomy was done. In the first five years more than 90 percent of men will have sperm in their ejaculate after reversal, but the rates drop steadily over the years. Two types of microsurgery are commonly used, and it's very important to find an experienced surgeon for either. The cost ranges from about $4,000 to $8,000.

Vasovasostomy seeks to reconnect the ends of the severed vas deferens. It can be done as an outpatient procedure (using a general anesthetic) and costs a few thousand dollars. With an expert surgeon, about 90 percent of the sperm will return, although pregnancy rates are somewhat lower than usual. The reason is that after a vasectomy, two-thirds of men develop antibodies to sperm. This immune response seems to affect the sperm's ability to fertilize an egg. Treatments for antibodies are not yet well developed, although there are some experimental drugs.

When a vas deferens has grown over too thoroughly for reconnection (one of the effects of time), it may be preferable to connect the downstream vas directly to the epididymis using a technique called vasoepididymostomy. This approach produces sperm in the ejaculate about three-quarters of the time, but pregnancy rates are somewhat lower than for vasovasostomy, probably because on average more time has elapsed since the vasectomy. In various studies, pregnancy has been achieved between 10 and 56 percent of the time.

When neither approach to vasectomy reversal is successful, a couple can still resort to an assisted reproductive technology, in particular ICSI.

Giving Birth Together

Once you've become pregnant, your partner should become a vital part of gestation and child birth. He should attend all your prenatal examinations so that he becomes knowledgeable about your nutritional and health needs during pregnancy and understands how events will unfold. There's nothing like the sound of the fetal heartbeat or the image on a sonogram to make the pregnancy real for him!

Likewise, you should attend childbirth education classes together. Most expectant fathers are considerably nervous about the prospect of being on hand at birth. Childbirth education relieves that. You'll both learn about exercises you can do before and during labor, how labor unfolds, the timing of contractions (something he should do), and what he can do to make you more comfortable during labor. He'll also be better prepared for your postpartum blues, which can be distressing to both of you. If the baby will be breast-fed, he should learn the reasons why so that he'll be supportive. Although you are the one with the equipment for that job, he can still participate. For example, he can bring the baby to you during the night or can change the baby afterward. This is only the beginning of a lifetime of ways he can be a caring, involved father.

The worst thing that can happen to a man before, during, or after his baby is born is to feel useless. Particularly with a first child, your partner can go from being the center of your attention to being a spectator. The last thing you want is a moody guy around the house. The more he can become part of the process, the better for everyone.

19

Mastering Midlife

For a woman, menopause is obvious. Whether menopause is easy or difficult, whether you have hot flashes or just stop menstruating, it's clear you're entering a new phase in your life. The physical cause of menopause is equally clear: a drop in the hormones estrogen and progesterone.

For a man, midlife changes are much subtler. Nonetheless, as my friend Gail Sheehy, author of *Passages* and *New Passages,* has noted, men do experience significant changes as they enter middle age. Their changes in hormone levels, while not as dramatic as women's, can affect mood, libido, energy, strength, bone density, and other physical characteristics. Most men not only fail to understand what's happening to them but consider the changes personal failures. You would never attribute a hot flash to your own inadequacies, nor would you tell yourself that "real women" don't get osteoporosis.

For men the biggest physical changes are a slower metabolism and less muscle—unless they exercise. These changes come from too much time sitting on the couch with a bag of potato chips. These changes will cause him to gain weight, which in turn increases the risk of all sorts of health problems. A young man can get away with gross neglect of his body, but a man at the far end of his forties can't. A healthful diet and regular exercise can make an older man feel twenty years younger.

When she was asked when midlife begins, my colleague Ruth Jacobowitz, author of *150 Most-Asked Questions About Midlife Sex, Love, and Intimacy,* said, "Ten years after however old I am right now." Ruth is an avid exerciser who watches carefully what she eats; her husband, Paul, fits that description, too. They're both fifty-something. Whether you think they're postponing midlife or making the very best of it, they're succeeding by knowing what they face and what to do about it.

Male Hormonal Changes

As men grow older, nearly all have lower levels of four hormones: growth hormone, melatonin, dehydroepiandrosterone (DHEA), and testosterone. For most guys the levels stay high enough to maintain important functions. For some, changes in hormones cause problems.

Growth Hormone

The most significant drop is in growth hormone. Produced by the pituitary gland, this hormone not only makes adolescents grow but also increases muscle mass and decreases body fat during the adult years. The hormone level peaks around age thirty, then declines steadily. Unless a pituitary gland problem develops, however, there will usually be enough to get by *if* the man finds other ways to maintain muscles and limit body fat. Unfortunately, if he doesn't, he will grow weaker and fatter as he gets older. By age seventy he will have lost half of his muscular strength.

Can growth hormone be replaced, much as a woman might take estrogen replacement therapy? Growth hormone therapy helps children with underactive pituitary glands, and it has been approved by the FDA for the wasting that can accompany AIDS. There have been only a few small studies of growth hormone injections in elderly men, and the subjects had unusually low levels of growth hormone. The hormones increased muscle mass by a few percent and reduced body fat by perhaps 10 percent. Unfortunately, the men gained no strength and reported no improvement in their well-being. Side effects included fluid retention, joint pain, and carpal tunnel syndrome (compression of a nerve in the wrist). Interestingly, when growth hormone was added to a program of strength training, it had no additional benefit. Also, strength training alone did more good than growth hormone alone. At approximately $12,000 a year, growth hormone injections don't seem to be the silver bullet against aging. Weightlifting is a better bet, and exercise has other benefits.

Melatonin

Melatonin is another hormone that declines with aging, especially in countries prone to overeating, such as the United States. (Calorie restriction usually increases the production of melatonin by the pineal gland, which is located in the brain.) Medical science is far from understanding all its jobs. We do know that it's intimately involved with our daily sleep cycles, the circadian rhythm.

There's been a tremendous amount of hype about the benefits of melatonin supplementation, but only a little research (and that with animals—and with contradictory results). So far it's been scientifically documented only to help certain sleep problems. Elderly insomniacs with unusually low melatonin levels may benefit from supplements. Melatonin often helps initiate sleep and allows them to sleep more soundly, although the overall length of sleep is about the same. Melatonin has also been used with some success in treating jet lag since it can help reset the circadian rhythm to a new time zone.

Because melatonin is sold as a food product, not a drug, it is not regulated by the FDA. The dosage is usually too large and often different from that claimed. Even one pill from most health food store preparations is serious overkill. Because repeated use can produce tolerance and fatigue, more is not better. Also, because melatonin is involved in so many bodily functions, messing with it is potentially serious business. This is one case where I definitely would *not* say, "What the heck, it can't hurt. Give it a try."

DHEA

I'm even more cautious about supplementing DHEA. DHEA is the most abundant male hormone in young men, yet we know very little about its function. Some DHEA is converted into testosterone and estrogen, but it's not a major source of either hormone. DHEA hits its highest levels in a man's twenties and declines by 70 to 90 percent by the time he's in his sixties.

Statistical studies have suggested a link between low DHEA levels and risk of heart disease in men over fifty, but efforts to stave off heart disease with DHEA have produced contradictory results. Two small studies reported that it increased well-being and leg muscle mass. So far the only established (although still experimental) clinical use for DHEA is in treating lupus, although some doctors have prescribed it for chronic fatigue syndrome.

Proper dosage is tricky. Before beginning therapy it's necessary to have a blood test that costs $75 to $100, which most insurance won't cover. Then, unless your man can talk a doctor into prescribing it, he must depend on the reliability of an unregulated over-the-counter product. After starting the hormones he should have his blood retested to make sure the dose is really correct. The best way to take DHEA is to find scientists researching its effects and participate in the study.

The biggest concern about DHEA is that it may promote the growth of prostate (and breast) cancer. As you'll learn in the next chapter, prostate cancer responds to levels of androgens in the blood. So it's possible, although not proven, that DHEA could help an insignificant tumor grow into a serious cancer.

Testosterone

Last on the list of flagging hormones is the big guy, testosterone. Not many years ago it was the standard prescription for any man with a potency problem. It seldom worked. Men keep hoping that testosterone will be the solution to their problems, but it usually isn't, especially if they are young or middle-aged. After age forty, testosterone levels typically drift down about 1 percent per year, but most older guys still have plenty to get the job done. More isn't necessarily better with testosterone; there seems to be a certain minimum level above which everything works correctly.

How often is low testosterone a problem? One study found that 1 percent of men between twenty and forty have low testosterone levels (less than 320 nanograms per deciliter of blood). That number rises to about 7 percent of those between forty and sixty, 20 percent of those between sixty and eighty, and perhaps as many as 35 percent of those over 80. At the Male Health Institute we find that low testosterone levels are responsible for potency problems in only about 5 percent of our patients. For those men it can really help.

Your man should not jump into testosterone supplementation without considerable care. If he's considering it, he should have repeated testosterone blood tests (taken in the morning when testosterone is usually highest). He should also have a test for "free testosterone," which tells how much of the hormone is actually available to do its job (the rest is bound to other molecules). The ratio of free to total testosterone helps determine whether there is a problem. When testosterone is low, prolactin levels should also be checked since high levels of this hormone suppress testosterone and suggest the possibility of a rare brain tumor. I recently diagnosed a tumor in a thirty-two-year-old man who saw me for potency problems.

Before forging ahead with testosterone supplementation, I also look for other, more subtle signs of testosterone deficiency. Most men with low testosterone not only have a flagging libido but also lack energy, have profound insecurities, and are depressed.

Testosterone affects the growth of prostate (and breast) cancer, so there's an element of risk, particularly for older men. I am constantly amazed at the number of men I see who have been taking testosterone for several years with no benefit. Some of them end up with prostate cancer. Urinary problems caused by prostate enlargement may also be worsened by testosterone replacement therapy.

The risks don't stop there. Oral and injected testosterone have been implicated in liver damage. All forms can thicken the blood, raising the risk of stroke and other circulatory problems. Sleep apnea may develop or worsen in men taking testosterone, they may experience breast enlargement, and their HDL (good) cholesterol level may drop. Any man taking hormones should have liver, PSA, and general blood tests each month. The new patch applications may lessen these risks by avoiding spikes in testosterone levels. It's also important to note that testosterone supplementation is for life. There's no such thing as a jump start. With long-term use, the testes will shrivel, and the body will not produce testosterone even if supplementation ends.

When testosterone supplements are called for, they can do wonders. Not only will his sex drive perk up, but he'll feel more energetic and upbeat. He'll also enjoy some protection from osteoporosis and may lose some fat and gain some muscle. For men who really need it, testosterone can be something of a fountain of youth.

Proper dosing can be difficult. Supplements are taken by either a shot or a patch applied to the skin. (A gel should be approved soon.) His doctor will need to monitor his blood levels of testosterone to perfect the dosage and frequency. With shots the necessary interval is usually somewhere between two and three weeks. Typically, the older a man is, the less often he will need shots because older males don't metabolize testosterone as quickly as younger ones do.

Men who can use patches usually have an easier time getting the right dosage because the patch introduces small amounts of hormone steadily throughout the day, avoiding the big spike of an injection and its subsequent falloff. At present there are two types of patches: those for the scrotum (where testosterone is absorbed five times more rapidly than through normal skin) and those applied to the trunk or upper arm. Each must be replaced daily, and the skin must be shaved to ensure adhesion. The nonscrotal patches have the advantage of not increasing levels of another androgen called dihydrotestos-terone (DHT). Although further research needs to be done, there is some concern that high levels of DHT may increase the risk of prostate enlarge-ment or cancer. About 9 percent of men have to quit using the patches because of irritated skin.

No matter what sort of testosterone supplement a man receives, his prostate needs to be monitored carefully. A man over fifty should have a PSA test each month (with a baseline done before treatment starts), a digital rectal exam every six months, and liver and blood count tests each year. In general, testosterone supplements don't seem to have profound effects on PSA or prostate size, but data have been conflicting. The conservative approach is never to assume that an increase in PSA or an enlarged prostate is being caused by the testosterone treatment. More tests should be done to rule out a serious problem.

How Sex Changes Over the Years

Although most men maintain sufficient levels of hormones to be sexually active throughout life, male sexual response does change somewhat with age. As long as both of you understand these changes and that they vary a lot from person to person, you can adapt to and even enjoy them.

As he grows older, it will take more stimulation for his penis to become fully erect. When in his twenties, the wink of an eye can do the job. By sixty, many men require direct physical stimulation to get stiff enough for intercourse, and the erection won't aim skyward the way it once did. Fortunately, other things take longer as well. He will also reach orgasm more slowly. It may take longer to run a mile, but you'll both have longer to enjoy the scenery. In fact, he occasionally might not come at all—and not mind a bit. In his twenties, sex was a sprint to the finish; later in life the journey may be much of the fun.

Although not every man ages sexually in the same way, most have slightly less forceful spasms during orgasm and ejaculate a smaller volume. Nearly all men require more time to be ready for sex again after orgasm. What took fifteen minutes fifty years ago may take a day or two now.

Most couples have sex less often in their later years, but they still have sex. Masters and Johnson found that about three-quarters of men over sixty still have sex at least once a month, and a third of married men in that age category are enjoying life's simple pleasure at least once a week. There's no reason not to continue enjoying each other physically throughout your lives.

Managing the Mental Aspects of Aging

Although exercise, diet, and the proper levels of hormones help a man approach and pass through midlife with aplomb, there's more to growing older than just the physical aspects. When retirement looms, a man faces the most abrupt, and often biggest, psychological change in his life. Whether he's your partner or your father, understanding that shift can help you both survive it.

As many as fifty years ago he entered the workplace. Schooling was mixed with mowing lawns, then there were summer jobs, and eventually a full-time occupation. For twenty years he focused on getting where he wanted to be, then he began to define himself by his job.

Many men become even more focused on their jobs when they become empty nesters. During the years of child-rearing, his life had purpose beyond his job. There were diapers to change, then ball games to attend, then science projects to aid. Those years flew by in a whirl of activity. When the kids go off on their own, he may count more than ever on his career for identity. He may keep on ascending the ladder or begin to be nudged aside by younger men. Eventually he will face the inevitability of giving up his identity as a worker.

There are lots of ways to ease that transition. Some men keep right on working but at a reduced level. Attorneys, for example, may simply take on fewer cases. Other professionals become part-time consultants. Still other men find purpose in retirement by taking up a new part-time job or by volunteering. President Jimmy Carter, for example, still exercises his diplomatic skills on occasion and spends time building houses with Habitat for Humanity.

It helps a lot to have interests outside the workplace before retirement. A few men get by on golf alone, but most need a portfolio of activities to stay healthy, keep sharp, and be happy. While he's still in the workplace, encourage him to have hobbies and get involved outside of his job. Whether he takes up woodworking, goes birdwatching, or joins a choir, he needs to start shifting the focus of life before retirement day.

Above all he has to stay active. Over and over I hear, "I'm too old to do that sort of thing." Men have it backward: That sort of thing will keep them young. Activity will bring them vigor and health. I know a couple in their eighties who downhill ski and travel on horseback to remote jungle locations. At seventy he joined the local volunteer fire department and pitched in with carpenters to build their new house. These people stay young by acting as if they're young.

His mind will need to stay active, too. Just like the biceps or abdominal muscle, the brain needs regular workouts. Preliminary research has shown that board games, which involve both the mind and hand-eye coordination, are particularly good at keeping older folks sharp. When one group of laboratory rats was allowed to play with objects and another only watched, the brains of the playful rats— and only the playful rats—actually grew in size. The key seems to be participation rather than observation. Television doesn't qualify as brain work.

You can help each other stay healthy, sharp, and happy into your senior years. As the responsibilities of work and family fade, you can truly enjoy each other. Instead of boarding one of those Sun City buses where nine out of ten passengers are women, you can ride off with him into the sunset.

I once struck up a conversation with a man in his early seventies. He was bouncing around the breakfast buffet of a motel where everyone, including him, was getting ready for a day of biking on a state trail. He and his wife were all decked out in snazzy biking shorts and shirts. I remarked on his high spirits. "Ah," he said knowingly, "when the kids leave home and the dog dies, *that's* when life begins."

Part IV

"Stormy Weather"

20

Prostate Problems

For a thirty-something man, the walnut-sized gland called the prostate quietly goes about its business of producing a portion of the volume of semen. In later life the prostate doesn't seem to do much but cause trouble. Cancer is certainly the most frightening prostate disorder, but plenty of other problems can also make a man's prostate his worst enemy. With age, many men's prostate enlarges, squeezing the urethra and reducing urine flow. Prostate enlargement can ruin a man's sleep patterns, sabotage his sex life, and chain him to the restroom. If left untreated, enlargement can cause hemorrhoids and hernia, damage the bladder and kidney, or cause urinary retention, which is life-threatening. Another very common problem is prostatitis, infection or inflammation of the prostate, which is difficult to eliminate and can continue for decades.

In this chapter I'm going to go into some detail about the diagnosis and treatment of prostate problems. In part I've chosen to do this because most women, understandably, know very little about prostate problems. You'll find little guidance in most general health books, too. In part I'm going to go into detail because the odds are very high that your partner will experience a prostate problem sometime. One in four men develop prostatitis, more than half have some degree of difficulty with enlargement by age sixty, and a man who lives long enough is very likely to have prostate cancer. (As many as 70 percent of men over eighty have at least a tiny prostate cancer, although few die from it.)

Fortunately, in the last decade there's been much progress in diagnosing and treating prostate disorders. Now that medical research is finally receiving enough federal funds, more findings will be coming. The treatments I describe in this chapter are state of the art in 1998. By the time you read this, however, important new discoveries will probably have been made. You and your partner should use the following as a base of knowledge and then do additional research into treatments to be sure you're up to date. With both of you on the case, you have a good chance of keeping his prostate from taking over your lives.

Prostate Cancer

As with many health problems, his chances of beating prostate cancer are greatly improved if the problem is detected early, if he's in good health otherwise, and if he has your full support. Take, for example, Jack, a fifty-six-year-old airline pilot I diagnosed with prostate cancer several years ago. Jack's employer required him to have a physical exam every year. Fortunately for him, the exams included PSA blood tests. We discovered Jack's cancer early, when it appeared to be confined entirely to the prostate. I discussed the treatment options with Jack and his wife, Patty, noting that the confined tumor, his relatively young age, and his excellent physical condition made him a good candidate for surgery.

Going into surgery, Jack had two other things going for him, too. First, Patty was very supportive and upbeat. Over the years I've found that men with involved and encouraging partners get through surgery better and recover more quickly. Second, Jack's attitude about his illness was very good. He wasn't depressed or even angry; he was just anxious to get on with it and beat the cancer.

I removed Jack's prostate in a two-hour surgery and was pleased to find that the cancer was limited to his prostate gland. Jack spent three days in the hospital, fewer than usual, then took it very easy at home for two weeks. At two months he was exercising again, visiting men who were soon to have prostate surgery, and becoming a leader in the local prostate cancer support group. At six months he completed a triathlon. Six years later Jack's PSA remains at zero, and he and Patty are enjoying an active, happy retirement.

Lowering His Risk of Prostate Cancer

Of course the best approach to prostate cancer is to prevent it in the first place. To find ways to reduce men's risks, doctors are asking the questions: Why do men get prostate cancer? And why are more and more men getting it? In the twenty years from 1973 to 1993 the number of cases skyrocketed. One reason is that we became so much better at diagnosing it. That's good since prostate cancer detected early is prostate cancer that can be cured. However, better diagnostic tools can't account for all of the increase since deaths also increased during the same time in the United States—by 25 percent! Meanwhile, prostate cancer deaths in other countries remain lower—in some cases *much* lower—than in the United States.

Worldwide, different nations and races have similar rates (perhaps 30 percent after the age of fifty) of "latent carcinoma," microscopic prostate cancer, yet the chances it will develop into clinically significant cancer vary greatly. An African-American man has the greatest risk of prostate cancer on Earth—ten times as great as a Japanese man and nearly fifty times that of some Chinese groups. Is the difference linked to race or way of life? Tellingly, an African American has a much higher risk than a black African man. Researchers began to think that something in the American lifestyle or environment was causing the growth of prostate cancers.

Indeed, they found that Japanese and Chinese men who move to the United States greatly increase their risk of prostate cancer. Within a generation Japanese men who moved to Hawaii increased their risk four to nine times, and Chinese men who moved to San Francisco increased their risk by three to seven times. A likely reason is the change in diet. American men get about 40 percent of their calories from fat, whereas Japanese and Chinese men get about 15 percent of their diet from fat. This observation led to a significant amount of research into the association between dietary fat and prostate cancer. As research mounts, the connection seems stronger and stronger.

To date, fifteen of nineteen studies have found increased risk (from small to tripled) among men who eat the most dietary fat, especially saturated fat. A Harvard University study found that men who ate a great deal of red meat were two and a half times more likely to develop advanced prostate cancer than those who ate the least.

Another possible risk factor for prostate cancer is smoking. In 1997, after years of looking, investigators found a link between prostate cancer and smoking. Smokers don't seem more likely to get prostate cancer, but their prospects are considerably worse when they do. Deaths are 34 percent higher among current smokers than among men who have never smoked. We don't know why this is so, but perhaps smoking suppresses the immune system's ability to fight the cancer.

Factors that may actually help prevent a prostate cancer from growing include soybeans, sunlight, vitamin E, lycopene, and selenium. Soy products, staples of the Japanese diet, contain genistein, a compound that reduces PSA levels in men and inhibits tumor growth in laboratory rats.

Sunlight may help because it synthesizes vitamin D in the skin. Scientists who study the patterns of disease have known for some time that more men die from prostate cancer in regions that receive less sunlight. In the United States, for example, risks are higher in the Northeast than in the Southwest. Furthermore, some researchers have found low levels of vitamin D in older men with prostate cancer. No study, however, has shown that vitamin D supplements help, so the best approach may be a judicious amount of sunlight exposure, perhaps a half-hour a day.

One study found that vitamin E, an antioxidant, reduced the risk of prostate cancer by about a third. Because vitamin E also seems to protect against heart disease (and perhaps other cancers) and is relatively safe, a supplement of 400 to 800 units a day can't hurt.

Selenium, a trace mineral in soil, may protect against some cancers. At this point, watch for future research results.

Genetics definitely play a role in the risk of prostate cancer. Your partner's risk doubles if his father or brother had prostate cancer. If two immediate relatives have had it, his risk is five times greater. Three immediate relatives pushes it to eleven times. The risk is further increased if the father or brother developed prostate cancer before age fifty-five. As this is written, some preliminary results suggest that genes might be involved, but we cannot at this point test for them in humans, so the best course is to know his family health history and be extra vigilant about screening if his risk is high.

To sum up, your partner can reduce his risk of prostate cancer by lowering his saturated fats, stopping smoking, including soy products in his diet, taking a vitamin E supplement, and getting a half-hour of sunshine every day. Things he should be doing anyway!

Detecting Prostate Cancer

In the early stages, prostate cancer has no obvious symptoms. By the time the cancer causes noticeable trouble, it has probably spread beyond the prostate and become incurable. Prostate cancer does grow more slowly than some cancers, but once it has spread, half of men will die within three years, so it's important to find it early when it's curable, through a combination of a digital rectal exam and a PSA blood test.

Your man should have a digital rectal exam (DRE) every year beginning at age forty and a blood test for PSA every year from age fifty (earlier for men with increased risk) to age seventy. As explained in chapter 4 on routine checkups, PSA is a substance made only by the prostate, and elevated levels suggest either cancer or another prostate problem. PSA is a far more effective test for prostate cancer than a rectal exam, but the latter does tend to catch cancers that PSA misses. Used alone, though, a rectal exam misses 30 to 40 percent of cancers, and most of the ones it finds are too advanced for effective treatment. PSA detects most cancers four to six years earlier than a DRE, and most of them are curable. Regular tests for PSA virtually eliminate unsuspected advanced prostate cancer.

Nonetheless, routine PSA testing is still controversial. Because the test detects cancer so well, some investigators have expressed concern that cancers will be treated that never would have caused problems. Critics point to the significant increase in prostate cancer surgery since PSA became widely used. In addition, PSA testing is expensive on a national basis. Supporters and recent studies say that regular PSA testing, when used appropriately, detects prostate cancer at an early stage, saves lives, and doesn't result in unnecessary surgery. They point out that PSA testing is no more expensive than mammograms and is better at detecting the cancer it's designed to find. I believe that the schedule in the preceding paragraph is prudent, and it is recommended by the American Cancer Society.

An elevated PSA reading or even an abnormal DRE doesn't necessarily mean cancer. Prostate enlargement, infection, or even recent ejaculation can elevate PSA, and nodules found during DRE may be benign. One elevated PSA measurement is cause not for panic but for follow-up.

PSA is generally considered elevated if it is over 4 nanograms per milliliter, but a lower or higher level does not mean either a clean bill of health or cancer. For example, many urologists think that the definition of "normal" should rise somewhat with age. For example, it might be wise to investigate further if a man in his forties and of high risk has a PSA over 2.5 ng/ml. If he were seventy, 6.5 ng/ml might be acceptable. Since black men have a higher risk of the cancer, a lower level should be investigated. As a rule of thumb, a PSA level between 4 and 10 ng/ml suggests a risk of cancer of 20 to 50 percent, between 10 and 20 ng/ml raises that to 50 to 75 percent, and above 20 ng/ml, 90 percent or greater.

Normal PSA Levels

AGE	NOT BLACK	BLACK
40–50	less than 2.5 ng/ml	less than 2 ng/ml
50–60	less than 3.5 ng/ml	less than 4 ng/ml
60–70	less than 4.5 ng/ml	less than 4.5 ng/ml
70–80	less than 6.5 ng/ml	less than 5.5 ng/ml

I can't tell you which number *your* man should use as a cutoff for going ahead with a biopsy. He should weigh the findings with his doctor, and both of you should discuss them. I can give you one hard number, though: About 25 percent of men with PSA readings between 4 and 10 turn out to have prostate cancer. Above 10 the odds of cancer rise sharply. I've tested men with PSA levels in the thousands.

If your man has a suspicious PSA measurement, further tests and calculations can check it out. If the level is between 4 and 10, the first step is to repeat the test since levels can vary as much as 45 percent from test to test. Then, if there have been previous tests, his doctor can compare the new reading to earlier ones to determine the "PSA velocity." When PSA increases faster than 0.75 ng/ml a year, cancer is likely. There has to be a baseline of at least three measurements taken over at least eighteen months.

Blood work may be done to analyze how much of the PSA is free (unbound to protein) in the bloodstream and how much is bound to proteins. For readings from 4 to 10 ng/ml, the free PSA should be at least 25 percent. If it is, there is a 90-plus percent probability that the PSA rise is caused by enlargement. This test can help determine whether a biopsy should be done.

A transrectal ultrasound can determine the size of the prostate so the doctor can do a "PSA density estimate." This test is often done when the PSA levels are between 4 and 9 ng/ml. The PSA reading is divided by the volume of the prostate in cubic centimeters. A result higher than 0.15 suggests a high risk of prostate cancer. This is an outpatient procedure that takes less than twenty minutes. While the man lies on his side, the doctor gently inserts a probe about the diameter of a finger into his rectum and then gradually withdraws it while the ultrasound machine provides an image of the prostate.

Ultrasound equipment is also used if there is a biopsy. It guides the placement of needles that remove samples of the prostate. In most cases there are six samples in a particular pattern, although suspicious areas noticed in a DRE will also be sampled. It's very important that these samples be taken from precise locations because cancer is much more likely to occur in some parts of the gland than others. About 85 percent grow in the muscular peripheral zone, and the other 15 percent start in the transition zone between the peripheral zone and the glandular zone toward the middle. Cancer rarely occurs in glandular tissue. A needle biopsy causes some discomfort, and there may be a little blood in his stool and ejaculate afterward. Antibiotics given before and after reduce the risk of infection, and the procedure is quite safe. Results are available in three to five days. It is always a good idea to have two pathologists examine the tissue. If the biopsy is negative but the PSA remains elevated, there should be another biopsy.

Most of the other tests his doctor might suggest are intended to show the extent of the cancer. Blood is routinely checked for elevated levels of acid phosphatase, which suggest spread of the cancer. In many cases a bone scan, in which a radioactive dye is injected, may be done to see if the cancer has spread to bones. Most doctors don't order a bone scan when the PSA is less than 10 ng/ml since the chance of a positive reading is only about 0.5 percent. There's no sense operating on a man if the cancer has spread to the bone since the surgery won't cure him.

A new test called ProstaScint reveals the spread to lymph nodes and other sites. It tags something called prostate-specific membrane antigen with a radioactive isotope that can be picked up during scanning. If the urologist suspects the local spread to the lymph nodes, he may also recommend computed tomography (CT), an imaging technique, or laparoscopic biopsy of the lymph nodes.

Being developed now are genetically based tests that will identify exceedingly small quantities of various prostatic cells in the wrong places. For example, reverse transcriptase-polymerase chain reaction-PSA and a similar test called RT-PCR-PSM (prostate-specific membrane globulin) can detect one metastatic prostate cell among one million blood cells. They should be very useful in detecting the spread of prostate cancer.

Prostate Cancer Staging and Grading

With the information from all these tests, doctors can describe the stage of the cancer by either the Whitmore-Jewitt or the Tumor, Node, Metastases (TNM) system. Both systems rate the cancer according to its size and extent, information that's crucial for choosing a treatment and predicting survival. Whitmore-Jewitt uses the letters A through D, with subdivisions for A and B. In the TNM system, the categories are T1 through T4, with subdivisions. TNM has two more descriptive letters: N for spread to the lymph nodes and M for distant metastases. The meanings of various stages are shown in the sidebar.

Physicians also assign a tumor a grade, which shows how aggressive it is. The Gleason score, assigned by microscopic examination of the biopsy, ranks the degree to which cells have lost their normal shape and configuration, a measure of malignancy. Cells that retain a normal appearance are said to be well differentiated, and those that have become masses are said to be undifferentiated. Because a Gleason score is the total of two measures of 1 to 5, it can never be lower than 2. Scores of 2 to 4 indicate a minor tumor that

Tumor, Note, Metastases and Whitmore-Jewitt Staging Systems for Prostate Cancer

TNM	W-J	DESCRIPTION
T0		No evidence of prostate cancer
T1a	A1	Found in surgery for benign tumor, less than 5 percent of tissue
T1b	A2	Found in surgery for benign tumor, more than 5 percent of tissue
T1c	B0	Detected by PSA, not DRE
T2a	B1	Involves half or less of one prostate lobe
T2b	B1	Involves more than half of only one prostate lobe
T2c	B2	Involves both lobes of prostate
T3a	C1	Extension from prostate on one side
T3b	C1	Extension from prostate on both sides
T3c	C2	Invading one or both seminal vesicles
T4a	C2	Invading bladder neck, sphincter, or rectum
T4b	C2	Invading additional areas adjacent to prostate
N0		No lymph node metastasis
N1	D1	Metastasis in single lymph node, 2 centimeters or less
N2	D1	Metastasis in single lymph node, 2–5 centimeters, or multiple lymph nodes
N3	D1	Metastasis in lymph node greater than 5 centimeters
M0		No distant metastasis
M1	D2	Distant metastasis

may just need to be closely watched. A score of 5 to 7 suggests that the tumor will grow and demand immediate attention. When scores rise between 8 and 10, the tumor is very aggressive and a surgical cure is in question.

Considering Surgery

One of the most difficult parts of dealing with prostate cancer is choosing a treatment method. Each approach has advantages and disadvantages, and there is never only one option. The best choice depends not only the stage of his cancer and its Gleason score but also on his age, his health (for example, heart disease), and his and your inclinations. The more you both know about the options, the better your chance of choosing the one that is right for him. The main choices are surgery, watchful waiting, radiation, and hormonal treatment.

The Partin Tables: Predicting Whether Cancer Is Confined to the Prostate

Alan Partin and his colleagues at Johns Hopkins University have developed this table to help men and their doctors estimate the likelihood that a tumor is confined to the prostate. It combines the information gained from the PSA, Gleason score, and staging. In the chart each number under "stage" shows the percentage of cancers likely to be confined to the prostate. For example, if the PSA is between 4.1 and 10.0, the Gleason is 5 and the stage is T1b, the probability is 70 percent.

		PERCENTAGE AT EACH STAGE						
PSA	GLEASON	T1A	T1B	T1C	T2A	T2B	T2C	T3A
0–4	2–4	100	85	92	88	76	82	—
	5	100	78	81	81	67	73	—
	6	100	68	69	72	54	60	42
	7	—	54	55	61	41	46	—
	8–10	—	—	—	48	31	—	—
4.1–10.0	2–4	100	78	82	83	67	71	—
	5	100	70	71	73	56	64	43
	6	100	53	59	62	44	48	33
	7	100	39	43	51	32	37	26
	8–10	—	32	31	39	22	25	12
10.1–20.0	2–4	100	—	—	61	52	—	—
	5	100	49	55	58	43	37	26
	6	—	36	41	44	28	37	19
	7	—	24	24	36	19	24	14
	8–10	—	11	—	29	14	15	9
>20	2–4	—	—	33	20	7	—	—
	5	—	—	24	32	—	3	—
	6	—	—	22	14	1	4	5
	7	—	—	7	18	4	5	3
	8–10	—	—	3	3	—	2	2

Surgery is appropriate only when the cancer is confined to the prostate. Despite the impression you probably got from all the previous discussion about staging, this isn't an easy thing to figure out without going in and looking. Even with the aid of CT scans and magnetic resonance imaging (MRI), we cannot tell absolutely unless we operate. Unfortunately, if the surgery determines that the cancer has spread beyond the prostate, the cancer will most likely return. To be a good candidate for surgery, the man also has to be otherwise healthy and young enough to have a life expectancy of at least ten years.

The most aggressive surgery, **radical prostatectomy,** removes the entire prostate. This procedure has been done since the turn of the century, and, frankly, when I first got out of medical school, it was unpopular for some good reasons: urinary incontinence and impotence. Now, however, most surgeons use a technique developed by Patrick Walsh at Johns Hopkins University, in which the surgeon carefully works around structures and nerve bundles. The risk of severe incontinence has been reduced to between 1 and 3 percent, and impotence to 40 to 50 percent. (For the latter complication it may take as long as a year to regain function, although some research suggests that early treatment with an erection medication, alprostadil, returns function sooner and more thoroughly.) Still, radical prostatectomy is serious surgery, requiring a surgeon with considerable skill and judgment. Not only must the prostate be removed without disturbing other tissues or nerves, but the urethra must be reattached to the bladder neck. Besides incontinence and impotence, possible complications include rectal injury (less than 1 percent), infection in 1.5 percent, lymph problems (swelling of a leg or legs) in 3.4 percent, and strictures (scarring of the urethra) in 6.7 percent.

If the cancer has been staged as T2b or above on the TNM scale or has a high Gleason score, the surgeon will probably want to sample a lymph node beforehand or at the beginning of the prostatectomy; if the lymph biopsy proves positive for cancer, the rest of the surgery may be canceled. Nonetheless, although the chances for a surgical cure decline with higher stage and Gleason score, men with stages as high as T3a and Gleason scores of 8–10 have been successfully cured by surgery.

After prostatectomy you can expect your partner to spend up to five days in the hospital. He'll have a catheter in place to drain urine for two to three weeks while the surgically rebuilt urinary tract heals. It will take him a few months to be his fully active self again, but the rewards can be significant. When the cancer really turns out to be localized, only about 3 to 11 percent of men (depending on stage) have some recurrence in the first five years, and only 30 percent after ten years. Even when postsurgical examination of the removed tissue suggests that not all the cancerous material could be removed, only about 50 percent of men with localized (near the prostate) cancers see their disease progress.

Watchful Waiting

At the other end of the spectrum from surgery, the least invasive choice is watchful waiting. This may be appropriate for men whose PSA and Gleason score suggest a confined tumor, particularly older men who wouldn't expect to live more than another ten years anyway. Although prostate cancer can be deadly, it usually advances fairly slowly, doubling in size every two to four years.

Watchful waiting consists of regular monitoring—PSA and DRE every six months and biopsy annually—to see if the cancer makes a move. If it does, further treatment can be chosen. Research has shown that men with low-grade tumors have a 90 to 94 percent chance of surviving ten years no matter what treatment is chosen, including watchful waiting. If the tumor is higher grade, watchful waiting's success drops to 45 percent. The advantage of watchful waiting is that it avoids the possible complications of more aggressive approaches, which can include bowel, urinary, or sexual problems. The disadvantages are that the cancer may spread and that the man will be older and less healthy if he needs aggressive treatment later on.

To be honest, most of my patients opt for treatments more aggressive than watchful waiting because they want to do *something*. Simply sitting around to see if they become more ill isn't very appealing. If watchful waiting is a good approach, the man may feel better if he pursues nutritional intervention—in other words, changes his diet to help fight the cancer. Although trials on diet and prostate cancer are only beginning, it makes sense that diet can make a difference. Since men all over the world have similar levels of latent prostate cancer but men who eat a lot of fat are more likely to develop significant prostate cancer, why shouldn't cutting dietary fat help slow cancer growth? Currently there is a study of a diet with less than 20 percent of calories from fat, along with a supplement of vitamins A, E, and D, and soy products.

Radiation Therapy

Radiation can be used to treat prostate cancers regardless of stage and for different purposes. It might be a first-line treatment at any stage, or it might be used when there is recurrence after surgery. Radiation can be applied externally by focusing beams on the tumor, or internally by placing pellets containing radioactive material (iodine-125 or palladium-103) directly in the cancerous area.

No studies have compared the results of surgery and radiation on patients with confined prostate cancers (T1 and T2), but evidence suggests that at least over five-year periods they achieve similar results. There is great controversy, however, over whether radiation remains as effective as surgery by ten years. In any event, radiation is a good option for an older man with a T1 or T2 tumor who might not tolerate surgery well. Conformal therapy (see below) may be a particularly good choice for locally advanced cancers (T2c). Radiation can also be useful for advanced disease to control the size of metastatic tumors, to combat local recurrence after prostatectomy, and to reduce pain and the risk of fracture when prostate cancer invades bones.

External beam radiation is usually applied five days a week for about eight weeks. Each sessions lasts less than ten minutes and involves no pain. Side effects include irritation of the urinary tract and bowels, both of which usually disappear over time. Incontinence occurs in less than 2 percent of patients. Impotence varies between 40 and 60 percent depending on the man's condition before therapy.

The implanting of radioactive seeds, called interstitial brachytherapy, can be done as an outpatient procedure under a mild general or spinal anesthetic. Ultrasound and a computer allow the doctor to place the seeds (smaller than a rice grain) accurately. Used alone it's most appropriate for early stage disease (T1c or T2a), Gleason scores under 7, and PSA less than 10. In other situations the radiologist may recommend pellets as an addition to external beam radiation.

Interstitial brachytherapy is too new—particularly the type guided by ultrasound imaging—for medical science to have good measures of outcomes. Early results are very encouraging at seven years after treatment, but physician experience and skill are very important. I await reports at ten and fifteen years to form a full opinion. It does appear, however, to have a lower risk of impotence than external beam radiation.

The latest technique for external beam radiation is called conformal radiation, which uses computer tomography and three-dimensional application to focus the beam closely on the tumor so more radiation can be applied without increasing side effects. At this time conformal therapy is available at academic institutions.

Hormonal Therapy

By eliminating or sharply reducing the hormone testosterone in the bloodstream, we can temporarily reduce the size of a prostate cancer or slow its growth. However, because some cells in prostate cancers are not affected by testosterone, the cancer will eventually grow. Though hormone therapy does not cure prostate cancer, it can reduce pain and add years to the life of a man whose cancer is beyond a cure by surgery or radiation. The effects are significant: A man who might have only a year or two without treatment often lives eight or ten years with hormonal therapy.

Testosterone can be withdrawn by removing the testes or taking medications. Either treatment causes impotence about 90 percent of the time and almost always causes loss of sex drive. Furthermore, there can be tenderness and swelling of the breasts, weight gain, loss of muscle mass, and osteoporosis. These are significant side effects, but I've known many men who lived a number of happy years thanks to hormone therapy after being diagnosed with advanced prostate cancer.

Although the approach sounds simple enough, choosing between the options isn't. Surgical castration is the cheapest approach (at about $2,000). It can be done as an outpatient, and recovery is easy. It is final, though, and many men have emotional issues with the prospect.

Pharmaceutical approaches to stopping testosterone production can be broken into two basic groups: estrogen and leutenizing hormone-releasing hormone (LH-RH) analogs. Diethylstilbesterol (DES) is the most widely used estrogen. DES blocks the release of something called leutinizing hormone from the pituitary gland, which stops the testes from producing testosterone. DES is taken orally once a day. The most significant side effects from DES are increased risk of circulatory problems such as heart attack, blood clots in the lungs, inflamed veins, and swelling of the legs. For that reason it's not appropriate for a man with heart problems. DES can also cause breast swelling and impotence, but it causes hot flashes in only about 11 percent of men.

LH-RH analogs replace the hormone that stimulates the release of the leutinizing hormone from the pituitary gland. Initially, LH-RH analogs cause a flare of testosterone, which needs to be controlled with antiandrogen for two or three weeks. Side effects include the familiar impotence, loss of libido, hot flashes, weight gain, lack of energy, loss of muscle mass, and osteoporosis. These drugs don't have such a negative effect on the circulatory system, however, and cause less breast enlargement. They're delivered as a monthly injection and cost $4,000 to $5,000 a year.

Another pharmaceutical approach to nullifying testosterone is to stop it from affecting cells. Antiandrogens bind to androgen receptors within cells, preventing testosterone from reaching them. Antiandrogens are used in the early stages of LH-RH therapy. Continuing them to block adrenal androgens doesn't appear to be more effective than LH-RH analogs alone. Research is being done into their combination with finasteride (Proscar), a medication for prostate enlargement (see below). The main advantage of antiandrogens is that they preserve potency in about 87 percent of patients. Hot flashes, diarrhea, and (rarely) liver problems are side effects.

Hormone therapy may also be used in other ways and in combination with other treatments. Intermittent androgen suppression, for example, uses an LH-RH analog (and sometimes an antiandrogen) until PSA drops, then continues it until PSA starts to rise again. The theory is that intermittent therapy reduces the growth of androgen-insensitive cells, prolonging the period that hormonal therapy is effective. No evidence yet exists that this works in human beings, but animals lived 50 percent longer when treated intermittently rather than continuously.

Other Promising Treatments

Cryotherapy, freezing the prostate, has actually been in use for a very long time, but modern techniques, which are a significant advance, have a track record of only about seven years. Cryotherapy has been used to treat confined cancers, where its effect is about the equivalent of surgery or radiation at five years. It has also been used to treat tumors that recur near the location of the prostate after surgery but not at distant sites. Modern cryotherapy hasn't been used long enough to demonstrate that it works as well as surgery or radiation. We'll know in ten to fifteen years.

Cryotherapy passes one or more probes through the perineum into the prostate, through which liquid nitrogen can be circulated to freeze the prostate. A catheter with warm circulating fluid prevents the urethra from freezing. The freeze-thaw cycle may be repeated to ensure that the cancer cells are killed. A man can expect to spend a couple of days in the hospital.

Although cryosurgery may be a less involved surgical procedure than prostatectomy, it, too, has complications. Varying with the hospital and doctor, impotence has occurred in between 41 and 86 percent of patients, incontinence has affected between 3 and 19 percent, and tissue sloughing (loss of dead tissue through the urethra) has caused problems in between 9 and 19 percent. A variety of other less common conditions, such as urinary retention, fistula (openings) into the rectum, and infections are possible.

At this point cryosurgery shows promise, but as the variation in side effects shows, it is a high-tech procedure that requires the right equipment and skilled doctors. Your partner should talk to his doctor about it and see how things have developed. It may or may not be a good choice.

Many other exciting treatments are on the horizon as I write this. Vaccines, monoclonal antibodies, and combinations of chemotherapy are under trial at major research centers. Keep an eye on the World Wide Web sites and publications of organizations such as the National Cancer Institute (800-4CANCER), the American Cancer Society (800-ACS-2345), the American Foundation for Urological Disease (800-242-2383), and major cancer centers such as Johns Hopkins, the Mayo Clinic, UCLA Medical Center, Massachusetts General Hospital, the Cleveland Clinic, Duke University Medical Center, Barnes-Jewish Hospital, Stanford University, Baylor University Medical Center, and Memorial Sloan-Kettering Cancer Center. There almost certainly will be important new developments by the time you read this.

Pain Relief

Even when therapy fails, it's important to understand that there are still ways to relieve pain and maintain as normal a life as possible. There is no reason for a man with terminal prostate cancer to be in pain. Conventional options are nonsteroidal inflammatory drugs, corticosteroids, morphine, and other narcotics. Recently the FDA also approved a drug called mitoxantrone (Novantrone) for use in combination with prednisone to treat pain from metastatic prostate cancer. Other choices are external beam radiation for bone pain, bisphosphanate drugs, and injections of strontium-89. For urinary problems caused by tumors growing in around the urethra, the standard surgical treatments for prostate enlargement that are described in the next section can help.

Prostate Enlargement

Benign prostatic hyperplasia (BPH) is a medical term mouthful, but it does a fine job of describing the problem. It is benign (not malignant, like cancer) hyperplasia (unchecked cell growth) in the prostate—in other words an enlarged prostate. BPH is a tumor, but it doesn't have the potential to spread outside the prostate.

Unlike cancerous prostate tumors, the nodules grow in the glandular tissue toward the middle of the prostate. Therein lies the difficulty. As the tissue grows, it pushes in on the urethra, restricting urine flow. In some men the muscular cells distributed throughout the prostate contract inappropriately, constricting the urethra. Thus some men with very large prostates may not have problems, but some with relatively small prostates but contracted smooth muscles may have a great deal of difficulty.

We don't know all or even many of the reasons that some men develop large or contracting prostates and others don't. Once again the problem is more common in Western than in Eastern countries, but in this case there's no strong evidence that dietary fat is a contributing factor. Genes, however, do seem to make a difference. One recent study found that when a man under the age of sixty-five has a very enlarged prostate, his male relatives are four times more likely to need BPH surgery sometime in their lives, and his brothers are six times more likely to need it.

In any event when the prostate squeezes the urethra, a chain of problems can develop. Because there's more resistance to urine flow, the bladder must contract more forcefully to push the urine out. This can thicken the walls of the bladder and decrease its capacity. The bladder can also become stretched out and lose its ability to contract effectively. As the urethra becomes more restricted, the bladder may not be able to empty completely. The poor owner of this enlarged prostate has to urinate more and more often with less and less success.

Men with prostate enlargement may experience a variety of symptoms, but the most common in one study were having to push (26.5 percent), difficulty starting urine flow (31.7 percent), incomplete emptying (31.7 percent), having to go twice or more during the night (36.8 percent), weak stream (40.2 percent), interruption of flow (40.5 percent), urgency (42.5 percent), and dribbling (46.4 percent). Overall, 51 percent of the men reported that their symptoms interfered with at least one aspect of daily living.

Diagnosing BPH

Even more than with most medical problems, many men resist going to the doctor for help with BPH. I think that's because they think that surgery is the only option and that impotence is inevitable. If your man is in denial about his symptoms of BPH, let him know that there have been important pharmaceutical developments in the past few years. Many men who seek treatment early—especially before the urethral restriction causes bladder problems—do well taking a pill each day. Even as recently as 1990, I performed 100 to 150 prostate surgeries per year; today it's less than 1 a month.

An office visit to a urologist for prostate enlargement will include many of the same procedures and tests as any other exam. His history will be carefully noted, including when he started to have the problem, its frequency, his symptoms, whether he's had blood in his urine (suggestive of bladder cancer) or signs of infection, and his medications (some drugs, including common decongestants, can make prostate problems worse). It's helpful if he records how much he drinks and voids for twenty-four hours. You can help him prepare for the visit by writing down such observations together. You may be more aware of some things than he is, for example, of how often he gets up during the night to urinate.

He'll also have a basic physical exam to rule out other problems that could be causing the symptoms, including strictures, neurological problems affecting the bladder, stones, and infection. The doctor may also want to watch him urinate. A digital rectal exam can provide information about the prostate's condition and size (not to mention the possibility of cancer), and urinalysis may be the only laboratory test. If infection is suspected, a urine culture may also be done. (If he hasn't had a PSA test recently, that may also be recommended, although BPH itself can bump up PSA levels.)

Once the doctor has ruled out causes other than BPH, your man will be asked to fill out the American Urological Association's BPH Symptom Checklist, which I've included in the Share Sheets at the end of this book. This quiz allows him and his urologist to assess the severity of his symptoms, which suggests whether further testing and treatment are necessary. Hand your man the Share Sheet before he has the exam so he can start making observations and notes that will be invaluable at the examination.

With more severe or long-term BPH, a blood test for creatinine can determine whether the kidneys have been damaged. Other diagnostic tests might also be recommended. Uroflowometry, measurement of urine flow rate, is probably the most common test. A high flow rate suggests that the problem isn't obstruction and that BPH treatments aren't likely to help. In unusual cases a test may measure the pressure generated by the bladder muscle. Low flow with high pressure suggests an obstruction, and low pressure points toward a nerve problem.

Imaging studies with ultrasound or, less commonly these days, intravenous pyelogram are generally used only when there's blood in the urine, infection, kidney problems, previous urinary tract surgery, or stones. The same goes for cystoscopy, which generally is used only for difficult, repeat cases or before surgery. When it is called for, cystoscopy—viewing the bladder with a device that passes through the urethra and prostate—should always be done with a *flexible* scope. Your partner is justified in running for cover if someone approaches him with a rigid scope.

Twenty-five years ago it was easy to choose an approach to BPH simply because there were so few options. Today's impressive array of treatments makes the choice a bit more complicated but also much more pleasant. Unlike for prostate cancer, there's no reason to adopt aggressive treatment early on unless a man's symptoms are causing him a great deal of discomfort or acute health problems (retention, infection, or stones, for example). Instead, he can start with less invasive treatments to see if they'll do the job.

Watchful Waiting

For any man with mild BPH and a few moderate symptoms, watchful waiting is a good first choice. The Mayo Clinic found that the symptoms of three-quarters of patients with mild BPH grew no worse over three and a half years. The most significant symptoms to watch for are a decrease in the size and force of the stream and an increasing feeling of incomplete emptying. Getting up in the night, although frustrating, doesn't mean he has to be treated aggressively. Your guy should see his doctor at least once a year to check on his progress, and he should avoid certain tranquilizers and over-the-counter decongestants that can worsen the problem.

Pharmaceutical Treatments

Pharmaceutical treatments for BPH have emerged since 1990, and we're still learning a lot about how well they work and for which men. Studies suggest that they will reduce symptoms in between 30 and 60 percent of men. At this point there are two quite different approaches to prescription treatment, called 5-alpha-reductase inhibitors and alpha-andrenergic blockers.

Finasteride (Proscar) is a 5-alpha-reductase inhibitor that blocks the conversion of testosterone into another hormone, dihydrotestosterone, a major player in the prostate. Finasteride actually shrinks the size of prostates in some men, increasing urinary flow rate. One study found that two-thirds of men taking 5 milligrams a day experienced at least a 20 percent reduction in prostate size after one to two years. Finasteride appears to be most effective for men with significantly enlarged prostates (larger than forty cubic centimeters) and recently has been shown to prevent urinary retention (the inability to urinate).

Finasteride takes weeks to months to begin working and doesn't approach full effect until six months, sometimes longer. It must be taken indefinitely or symptoms will return. Impotence occurs in 3 to 4 percent of men who take finasteride, and it also reduces the volume of ejaculate. Breast enlargement is a side effect for a very small number of men; it's not known whether this might increase the risk of breast cancer. Finally, finasteride cuts PSA levels by at least 50 percent. For that reason a PSA test should be done before beginning the drug, and any subsequent test that doesn't drop at least 50 percent should be considered suspicious. Thereafter, the PSA results should be multiplied by two to get a more accurate reading. For this reason, it is important that he tell his family doctor that he is taking Proscar.

Alpha-andrenergic blockers were originally blood pressure drugs. They relax muscles in the walls of blood vessels. As it happens, they also relax the muscles in the prostate, helping with contraction problems. Although a number of these medications are available, the FDA has approved only doxazosin (Cardura), terazosin (Hytrin), and tamsulosin hydrochloride (Flomax) for treatment of BPH.

The trick with alpha blockers is getting the dose right. Most men respond best when receiving 4 to 5 milligrams per day (0.4 for Flomax), but some experience side effects at this dose, including low blood pressure (dizziness), fatigue, and headaches. It's generally best to start with a lower dose (2 milligrams) and work up until symptoms have been eliminated. The side effects can be reduced by taking the medicine in the evening. One significant advantage of alpha blockers is that they work almost immediately.

At a 10-milligram dosage of alpha blockers, one study found a 30 percent reduction in BPH symptoms in two-thirds of men. Another study found that 10 milligrams reduced American Urological Association Symptom Index scores from 20 to 12.4 (from the lower end of severe to the lower end of moderate symptoms). Other studies have found reductions in symptoms as great as 40 percent and urine flows that more than doubled. Side effects cause about 10 percent of men to discontinue the drugs. Alpha blockers are a good choice, too, for men who also have mild hypertension (blood pressure) since they help with that problem, too. (They don't usually lower blood pressure in men without hypertension.)

There is emerging evidence that finasteride and alpha blockers work better for different groups of men. Men with large prostates may benefit from the shrinkage caused by finasteride, whereas those with small prostates may benefit more from the muscle-relaxing effects of the alpha blockers. Nonetheless, since alpha blockers work sooner than finasteride and cost a little less, many urologists suggest trying them first.

An herbal preparation called saw palmetto has had limited clinical trials in the past few years. It's widely used in Europe to treat BPH. Most of those trials have shown some improvement of BPH symptoms, although the duration of the experiments was generally short. No one knows, however, how saw palmetto works. We don't know what effect saw palmetto might have on PSA levels, but it appears to have few significant side effects. Your guy might try it under the supervision of his doctor. Other herbal remedies, such as Pygeum africanum, pumpkin seeds, beta-sitosterol, and cernilton, have an even more limited track record for BPH. Whether they're helpful and safe remains to be determined.

Surgery for BPH

Surgical procedures for BPH are numerous. The most common, **transurethral resection of the prostate (TURP),** is the second most common surgery paid for by Medicare. At its peak at least 360,000 were done every year, although less aggressive procedures, including medications, have slightly reduced that number.

TURP has been referred to over the years as the "gold standard" because it relieves the symptoms of prostate enlargement most effectively. With the patient under anesthesia, the surgeon inserts an instrument called a resecto-scope through the urethra, then cuts away the inner part of the prostate with a wire (not the entire prostate, as in open prostatectomy). Among men with severe symptoms, 93 percent enjoy marked improvement.

Still, TURP may not be the answer for your partner. Although it's very effective, TURP also is the most expensive approach and has the highest complication rate short of open prostatectomy. (Open prostatectomy isn't often used for BPH, but it may be appropriate for especially large prostates.) Between 5 and 10 percent of men who have TURP become impotent, and 2 to 4 percent become incontinent. Nearly all men who have TURP will have retrograde (into the bladder) ejaculation. TURP also requires hospitalization for one or two days, about 6 percent of men require a blood transfusion, 10 percent will need a repeat surgery, and a catheter remains in place for one to three days. Recovery from TURP takes one to three weeks.

A close relative of TURP is **transurethral incision of the prostate (TUIP),** which makes two deep incisions instead of cutting away tissue. TUIP can be done more quickly than TURP, costs less, and works nearly as well, but it's only effective for men with relatively small prostates.

A host of other approaches are under development. **Balloon dilation,** for example, compresses prostatic tissues with an inflatable device at the end of a catheter. Balloon dilation can be done under local anesthetic as an outpatient and usually improves symptoms noticeably while producing few significant side effects. Over time, however, the effects dwindle, and the procedure must be repeated after about a year or a different therapy used. For that reason, it's not in such favor now.

Thermal treatments heat prostatic tissue to about 113 degrees Fahrenheit, either to damage nerves in the prostate that cause it to contract or actually destroy prostatic tissue. The heat may be applied by electrical resistance, microwaves, ultrasound, radio waves, or lasers. An FDA-approved microwave technique called the Prostaron is a choice for men with medium-sized prostates.

Another approach, **transurethral needle ablation (TUNA),** delivers low-energy radiowaves through small needles. TUNA and similar approaches can significantly relieve symptoms, at least temporarily, and the complications are minor, but treatment may have to be repeated. Time will tell how they work over the long haul.

High-intensity focused ultrasound (HIFU) destroys prostatic tissue while sparing nearby tissue. One trial has shown about a 50 percent improvement in symptoms and flow rates, although urinary retention was a problem in three-quarters of the men for a few days, and half had blood in their ejaculate for as many as three months. In one trial, most of the symptoms were still improved after two years.

Another way to selectively destroy prostate tissue is **lasers.** It takes one to three months for the destroyed tissue to slough off and open the way for urine. It's usually performed on an outpatient basis but may require a catheter for up to a week. In the long run it may turn out to work nearly as well as TURP.

The last method uses a **very powerful wire** to vaporize prostatic tissue instead of just cutting it away. Early results suggest that the procedure can be done on an outpatient basis with a catheter in place for only about twenty-four hours. How well the improvements last remains to be seen.

The emergence of new surgical approaches to treating BPH is very encouraging, but you and your spouse should bear in mind that they must prove themselves against the standards: TURP and TUIP. Only when they prove to be at least as effective with fewer complications should they be considered real alternatives. That's why I rarely use them.

Soothing the Savage Prostate

Whether your partner's prostate problems come from enlargement, infection, or other irritation, there's quite a bit he can do to make himself more comfortable. Suggest that he:

• drink eight glasses of water per day. Too many men cut back on fluids when they have prostate problems, assuming that they will reduce symptoms. Actually, diluting urine reduces symptoms, although he should increase his water intake gradually.

• avoid sitting for extended periods. He's sitting on his prostate, and it doesn't like it.

• get some exercise. Although we don't know why, regular endurance exercise seems to reduce prostate problems.

• avoid caffeinated beverages. Caffeine is a diuretic, causing the body to excrete fluids, making prostate problems worse.

• steer clear of alcohol. Booze worsens prostate problems in nearly all men.

• be careful of spicy foods and chocolate. For some men they irritate the prostate.

• try a hot bath. Sitting in warm water eases prostate symptoms for many men.

• ejaculate regularly. The prostate seems to respond negatively to an increase or decrease in frequency. That's a prescription he probably won't mind.

• try to relax. Relaxation techniques such as meditation help many men with problem prostates.

For men who wouldn't hold up well under a more aggressive treatment, there are also coiled plastic or metal springs called **stents** that can be used to hold the urethra open and allow urine flow. It takes only about fifteen minutes to place a stent, although it's tricky to get it in just the right place. There aren't long-term studies of their effectiveness, but so far they appear to work well and produce minimal adverse reactions.

Prostatitis

Prostatitis, inflamed prostate, is a category of prostate problems that many doctors would prefer to have never heard about and that some have even chosen to ignore. Indeed, some of the best published material on prostate cancer and enlargement fails to even mention prostatitis. Let me assure you, for men who have it, it's impossible to ignore. The problem is very real and very difficult to treat. They may suffer years of urinary discomfort, urgency, and frequency; they may have constant aches in their lower back, testes, or behind the scrotum; they may find ejaculation painful enough to give it up altogether. Perhaps the most shocking thing about the situation is how common it is. Some investigators have estimated that prostatitis is the most common prostate problem of all—affecting as many as half of all men at some time. However, the medical community is far from unanimous about what prostatitis is or what to do about it.

Acute bacterial prostatitis is the easiest form to diagnose and treat. An infectious agent—or at least white blood cells, a sign of infection or inflammation—is found in the urine or in prostatic secretions obtained by prostate massage. (Prostate massage is much like a digital rectal exam. The doctor inserts a gloved and lubricated finger through the man's anus and applies pressure and motion to the prostate through the wall of the colon.) A man with acute bacterial prostatitis usually has burning on urination and urgency, and may have discharge at the tip of the penis. Often he will also run a fever, and his prostate will be tender when examined by a digital rectal exam. The doctor will first rule out STDs, then prescribe a three- or four-week round of a quinolone antibiotic or another tailored to the organism. Some men will have another bout months or even years later. Acute bacterial prostatitis is less common than the other types, which aren't as easy to treat.

Chronic bacterial prostatitis also seems to be caused by bacteria, but it doesn't respond as well to antibiotics. About two-thirds of men with acute prostatitis don't respond completely to the first course of antibiotics, so most doctors extend the drugs for another six weeks, which helps about another third.

Overall, only about 5 percent of men with some form of prostatitis are cured by antibiotics alone. Of the remaining 95 percent, some are diagnosed as having chronic bacterial prostatitis but aren't cured by antibiotics. A larger group have some symptoms of inflammation of the prostate—tenderness and the presence of white blood cells—but no bacteria is found in their urine or prostatic secretions. Buckets of antibiotics don't seem to help. At this time, four answers have been proposed for these prostate problems that refuse to be pigeonholed.

According to an article in the *British Journal of Urology*, a doctor at a clinic in the Philippines thinks that bacteria or fungi cause many cases of chronic prostatitis but that they are not readily cultured by traditional techniques or killed by standard antibiotic protocols. He employs prostatic massages three times per week along with antibiotics in order to empty all prostatic ducts and allow antibiotics to access these places. Such techniques haven't been confirmed by rigorous trials, but there are numerous positive anecdotal reports from patients, and some U.S. urologists are experimenting with the practice. Indeed, some patients and their partners have been trained to do every-other-day massages at home. Treatment may last as long as four months depending on the results of cultures for organisms.

Researchers at the University of Washington used DNA techniques to examine biopsies of prostatic tissue from men with prostatitis and found previously unidentified bacteria in 77 percent of them. Whether these bacteria caused the men's symptoms is another question, but the study does suggest that it may be difficult to identify the organisms causing prostatitis.

Another theory is that prostatitis is an irritation caused by urinary reflux. A Swedish study found that prostatic secretions contained significant amounts of urine in about 25 percent of men with prostatitis. At the least, urinary reflux is a logical way for pathogens to make their way into the prostate and cause infection. Reflux may also cause chemical irritation. Furthermore, treatment of men with a drug that reduces the concentration of acid in urine cut pain in half.

Finally, some researchers believe that at least some cases of prostatitis are caused by an immune system reaction. A group from the University of Maryland looked at ways a type of immune cell called T cells reacted to proteins present in the prostate. They found elevated T-cell activity among four of fourteen men with nonbacterial prostatitis but in none of a group of fifteen control subjects. If further work confirms that some men may be having immune system reactions, immune system suppressants such as steroids might help.

A final category of prostatitis is what's routinely called prostatodynia—symptoms of prostate problems without any evidence of inflammation (white blood cells). Prostatodynia appears to be related to muscle tension in the prostate or the pelvic floor muscles. Alpha blockers such as terazosin (Hytrin) or doxazonsin (Cardura) often help men with prostatodynia since the medication relaxes those muscles. (This and other findings have led some to wonder if there's really a difference between prostatodynia—or even nonbacterial prostatitis—and BPH. In my experience there usually is.)

If this sounds like a pretty depressing analysis of the status of the most common disease of the prostate, there is good news. Through the work of groups such as the Prostate Foundation and the American Foundation for Urological Disease, prostatitis has been getting much more attention in the media, the medical community, and the government. In the fall of 1997 prostatitis was brought to the attention of the U.S. Congress, and there was debate about funding for research into the problem.

I'm hopeful that in five or ten years we'll look back on prostatitis much as we now look back on the bad old days of prostate cancer and BPH. For now, if your guy has fallen prey to prostatitis, I know it's a difficult thing to watch. Help him get involved—starting with a connection to the Internet, where he'll find active discussion groups of other men (and their partners) who are working out their prostate problems with each other's assistance. There's a supportive community out there; be sure he joins it!

21

Guy Troubles

Because of your monthly menstrual ritual and your annual Pap smear, you've become accustomed to the notion that things can go wrong in your urogenital tract, especially if you don't maintain it well. Furthermore, the odds are high that you've already had a urinary tract infection and are familiar with the importance of hygiene, antibiotics, and cranberry juice.

Men don't see things that way. They may know about the prostate and anticipate problems with it when they get older, but they otherwise expect flawless performance from their urogenital tract without a bit of maintenance. Unfortunately, although they may face fewer reminders than you do, they're going to be disappointed. Some men are healthier or luckier than others, but almost none escapes one of the problems we'll talk about in this chapter. From urinary tract infections to a hernia, something is going to catch him by surprise before old age does. Surprise is the key word. He'll be surprised it's happening, surprised it won't go away, and surprised he has to see a doctor.

Only by not knowing what's wrong and what should be done can a man continue to imagine that things will sort themselves out. Together we can cure some of that ignorance—and some men while we're at it.

Incontinence

More women than men are unable to fully control the release of urine, but the problem is far more common among men than most people (including medical professionals) imagine. In particular, temporary or (rarely) long-term incontinence often follows removal of a man's prostate. Too many men (and women) with continence problems have been offered nothing other than a recommendation to wear diapers or the option of surgery to rebuild the urethral sphincter. They may not even be told about the range of nonsurgical alternatives, and if they are, insurance companies may resist paying for them. That's a shortsighted approach since surgical correction is far more expensive.

The exercises called Kegels can improve the ability to control urine flow and strengthen the muscles of the pelvic floor. One technique for teaching Kegels is to stop and start urine flow repeatedly. Since this may be difficult to learn after prostate surgery, it's important that a man do Kegels *before* as well as after the surgery. It often seems helpful to do two kinds of Kegels: short, repeated contractions and longer ones lasting three to ten seconds.

Diet can also help with incontinence problems. Spicy or acidic foods are the most common culprits. He should eliminate them for ten days, and then

---

How to Do Kegels, Male Version

While women are often taught to do Kegel exercises by stopping the flow of urine, men learn the technique best a different way. The man should imagine trying to prevent gas from escaping from the anus. He should tighten and lift the rectal area without flexing the muscles of the buttocks or abdomen. At least at the beginning, he should check that the abdomen and buttocks muscles aren't flexing by watching in a mirror or feeling with hands. It may take some experimentation to isolate the correct muscles of the pelvic floor.

Once he's found the muscles, he can do two types of exercises. The first involves slowly tightening the pelvic muscles—drawing them up—and holding for five seconds at a time. At first he may not manage to hold them for five seconds, but after several weeks of practice, it will come. He should rest for ten seconds between exercises and repeat until the muscles become tired. The other exercise is quick contractions and releases. Again, repeat until the muscles become tired.

He can do the exercises practically anywhere and anytime—sitting at his desk, in the car, watching TV—and no one else will know.

Written and audiotaped instructions for learning Kegels are available from Help for Incontinent People (800-252-3337).

Foods That Can Irritate the Urinary Tract

Alcoholic beverages
Apple juice
Apples
Cantaloupe
Carbonated drinks
Chiles and other spicy foods
Chocolate
Citrus foods and juices
Coffee
Cranberries
Grapes
Guava
Milk products
Onions
Peaches
Pineapple
Plums
Strawberries
Sugar
Tea
Tomatoes
Vinegar
Vitamin B complex
Vitamin C (unless buffered with calcium carbonate)
Vitamin E (unless in powdered form)

add them, one at time, to see what he tolerates. Equally important, he should be drinking lots of water to dilute his urine.

A bladder can develop bad habits that lead to leaking and an unusual urge to urinate. Like a child who leaves the toilet seat up, that bladder needs to be trained to behave correctly. Believe it or not, to gradually increase bladder capacity and decrease frequency of urination, he needs to drink more water. He should drink at least a quart a day and gradually increase to two quarts. At first he may need to go more often, but eventually he'll be able to retain more of this diluted urine, which is less irritating to the bladder. When he gets the urge, he should try to hold it for five more minutes, and he should add five minutes a week. Within two to three months he should be able to hold up to 14 ounces in his bladder and urinate every two to four hours.

Other less frequently used behavioral approaches to taming incontinence include electrical stimulation of the pelvic floor muscles to strengthen them and biofeedback to help patients isolate and strengthen pelvic floor muscles. For men with mild or moderate incontinence, these approaches may be very helpful.

Men who are incontinent after prostate surgery have enjoyed some success using injections of Teflon or, more recently, collagen into the urinary sphincter. Depending on the method of prostate removal, injections can return full control to as many as 78 percent and improvement in another 10 percent. The FDA has approved collagen injections for treatment of incontinence but requires that urologists undergo training and certification for administering them.

Although the techniques I've just described may eventually solve the problem, he'll have to live with leakage in the interim. He may want to wear continence briefs, sold in drugstores. Pads that fit over the penis or attach to regular underwear may work for mild leakage. A "condom catheter" can keep a man with a serious problem dry. Various designs of penile clamps can also be used to stop leaks, but a man needs to use these with considerable caution and after having thorough instruction. Models with Velcro straps may be safer than the older Cunningham penile clamp.

Urinary Tract Infections

A urinary tract infection, caused by infectious agents such as bacteria passing up through the urethra, results in painful urination, irritation, frequent and urgent urination, and discharge at the tip of the penis. Differences in anatomy make simple urinary tract infections much less common for men than they are for women. His urethra is about four to six inches long, while yours is about one inch long, and yours is a lot closer to the anus than his is. If an infectious agent takes up residence in the male urogenital tract, it will probably pick the prostate or the epididymis instead of the urethra. Still, infection along the urethra and into the bladder is possible and needs to be treated to prevent further problems.

Frankly, most men who think they have a urinary tract infection turn out to have an STD, so his doctor will rule out that possibility first.

Can he catch a urinary tract infection from you? Yes, but it doesn't happen very often. Because of the male design, it's difficult for pathogens to make their way into the urethra. As is the case with your system, infection is even less likely if he urinates shortly after having intercourse. This basic precaution will do a lot to reduce the chances of a rebounding infection that's passed back and forth between sexual partners. If you or he develops a fungal infection, you should both be treated.

Epididymitis

Each year about half a million American men have a bout of epididymitis, an inflammation of the tubular masses on the back of the testes. Infection causes at least 80 percent of the cases. Among younger men, half the time the cause is chlamydia, with gonorrhea running second. In men over forty years of age, coliform bacteria from feces are more often to blame, although the sexually transmitted organisms are certainly a possibility.

How do such organisms make their way so far into the male urogenital tract? They're carried in urine that backs up through the vas deferens, called retrograde urination or urine reflux. In fact, in the roughly 20 percent of cases of epididymitis where no organism can be identified, it appears that the inflammation is caused by chemicals in the urine.

Epididymitis usually comes on fairly quickly, causing swelling, tenderness, and redness of the testes that peak within twenty-four hours. It can be quite painful and may also cause nausea and fever. Both sides of the testes become involved about 10 percent of the time. Anytime a man has severe pain in his testes, however, testicular torsion should be ruled out first, since loss of the testes is likely if it continues for more than six hours. (For more about testicular torsion, see chapter 18.)

There's no sense trying to wait epididymitis out. He needs to rule out torsion anyway, and prompt treatment reduces the risk of scarring and infertility. In rare cases a runaway infection can cause serious damage. If your partner shows symptoms of epididymitis, he should see a doctor right away. After a urine culture is done, he'll most often take an antibiotic appropriate to the organism involved. (If the organism is an STD, you'll be treated as well.) An over-the-counter pain medication such as aspirin or ibuprofen also helps, as will a supporter to take pressure off the spermatic cord. He should apply ice packs for the first forty-eight hours and then take hot baths.

Testicular Cancer

Urologists look with some pride at the strides made in successfully treating testicular cancer. The death rate has dropped more than 70 percent in the past twenty-five years, and 95 percent of men diagnosed today survive and live relatively normal lives. Only 350 American men died of testicular cancer in 1997, and nearly all of those deaths were unnecessary. Their cancers simply weren't detected early enough through that simple self-exam described in chapter 5. However, testicular cancer remains the most common solid cancer in males fifteen to forty-four, so every man should do the exam regularly, particularly younger men.

The self-exam is so important because testicular cancer often grows rapidly. The year or more that lapses between doctor visits can give it plenty of time to escape the testes and invade the lymph system or even the brain. A once-a-month check on his (or your) part is vital.

If cancer is detected early, the treatment is straightforward: remove that testicle. Most of the time, the tumor develops on only one side, so another perfectly fine testicle remains, providing plenty of sperm for fertility. If the loss of the testicle is emotionally distressing to a man, a prosthesis can closely match the remaining testicle.

Even when the malignancy has moved beyond the testicle, treatment is usually successful although more complicated. Sites to which the tumor has metastasized (to the lymph system, abdomen, or lungs, for example) may require surgery. Chemotherapy is usually in order, and radiation may be needed. In such instances, infertility is common—about 50 percent after chemotherapy.

The Various "Celes"

A hydrocele is an accumulation of fluids around the testes. Rare among adult men, the problem is very common in newborns. It may resolve itself. A hydrocele is painless and isn't a cause for medical concern in men, but a doctor should rule out the possibility that it has been caused by another problem, such as testicular cancer. We can usually make this distinction easily by shining a light at the scrotum. A hydrocele will be translucent, whereas a tumor will be opaque. (In boys a hydrocele may be difficult to distinguish from, and may be involved with, an inguinal hernia—see below—which requires correction.)

Most of the time we don't know what causes a hydrocele. Unless it produces discomfort, gets in the way, causes a bulge in his pants, or makes a testicular self-exam difficult, it's usually best to leave it alone. The fluid can be aspirated, but that opens the possibility of infection, and the hydrocele most likely will return anyway. Surgery can correct a hydrocele, but I don't recommend it for mild cases. If it's large, however, it may be embarrassing or get in the way.

Spermatocele, a collection of fluid in the epididymis, seldom causes problems and can usually be left alone. Many men have very small ones, rarely large enough to be noticeable. A man should be justifiably concerned about testicular cancer and have a doctor check the lump, but if spermatocele is the diagnosis, neither of you needs to worry about it. It has no effect on fertility and isn't cancerous.

Varicoceles are discussed in chapter 18 because they can affect fertility.

Urethral Stricture

A narrowed urethra can restrict urine flow, much like an enlarged prostate does. Males can be born with a narrowed place, called a urethral stricture, or it can be caused by infection, injury, or surgery. Strictures used to be more common than they are today because gonorrhea, the infection most likely to cause scarring and strictures, often went untreated. Today, antibiotics generally knock gonorrhea out before it does damage.

Strictures used to be treated by passing progressively larger flexible tubes through the urethra, gradually stretching it back to normal size over several months. Some evidence suggests that Benjamin Franklin used the technique on himself! In recent years, however, a small telescope-guided surgical device has been used to cut away the scar tissue with good success. In other cases a titanium springlike device called a stent can hold the urethra open.

Priapism

Most men imagine that a prolonged erection would be a dream come true. That's definitely not the case when that erection is unaccompanied by sexual feelings and persists for several hours, a condition called priapism. Any erection that lasts longer than four hours is cause for serious concern because it can cause permanent damage to the tissues of the penis. Immediate medical attention is in order. Causes are an overdose of a medication for potency problems, blood disorders, and prescription medicines. If your partner has erections in nonsexual situations or if his erection remains after ejaculation, he should talk to his doctor about it.

Problems of the Uncircumcised Male

I discussed the issues surrounding circumcision in chapter 13, but it's worth mentioning a few conditions that can develop in a man whose foreskin is intact. Most are rare and can be made less so by good hygiene, but they can become serious problems if uncorrected.

Balanitis

Balanitis is an inflammation of the foreskin. It can develop because of friction from damp clothing, chemicals used to clean clothing, or contraceptives such as latex condoms and contraceptive foams or jellies.

Phimosis

Phimosis, the inability to retract the foreskin during erection, can be congenital or can develop as the result of chronic infection. Your partner undoubtedly knew long ago whether the first condition applies, but the latter can develop and lead to the need for circumcision.

Paraphimosis

Paraphimosis is the opposite problem from phimosis: The foreskin retracts but then won't return back over the head of the penis. It can develop from infection or injury and needs to be dealt with promptly before swelling makes the problem worse. Often a lubricant will take care of paraphimosis, but circumcision is the permanent solution.

Inguinal Hernia

A hernia is the protrusion of an organ through an abnormal opening. The type that disproportionately affects men is called an inguinal hernia. About a quarter of all men will have one in their lifetimes, as opposed to only 2 percent of women.

There's a potential weak spot at the point where the spermatic cord from the testes passes through the pelvic floor and into the abdominal cavity. If the muscles at this spot deteriorate or become torn, the intestine can protrude through the abdominal wall into the groin or scrotum. Many people think that hernias are caused by straining or lifting heavy objects, but there often is no direct explanation for a hernia. They are, however, more common in overweight people.

The onset of a hernia may be gradual and not very painful. Men often feel a heaviness in their lower abdomen or groin. This may be more severe when bending over or coughing and may disappear when lying down. Eventually they notice a bump or protrusion in the groin or scrotum. If a hernia enters the scrotum, there is usually significant discomfort.

A protruding intestine needs to be returned promptly to the abdominal cavity in order to prevent strangulation of the intestine. The doctor may be able to push the intestine back into the abdominal cavity, and a truss may keep it there, but this doesn't correct the problem. Surgery is the only permanent cure. It is, in fact, the most common surgery done in the United States. More than 600,000 traditional hernia repairs are done each year. Fortunately, there have been many developments in hernia surgery over the past ten years.

Traditional hernia repair is called herniorrhaphy. The doctor makes an incision several inches long, pushes the organ back through the abdominal wall, and sews the torn or separated muscles together. Hernia surgery isn't difficult and has a high rate of success, but it does require at least an overnight stay in the hospital.

Hernioplasty was developed in the early 1990s and was initially used just for hernias that recurred after traditional repair. Today, however, it's often recommended for the initial work. During a hernioplasty, a synthetic mesh is placed over the damaged muscles to prevent organs from protruding. The mesh can be installed by a conventional incision or laparoscopically. In laparoscopy, the surgeon makes several small incisions and inserts tiny tools and a video device. The surgeon does the work guided by a video monitor rather than opening a large incision. Because laparoscopic hernioplasty involves such small incisions, recovery is usually quicker than with conventional surgery. It also can sometimes be done on an outpatient basis.

Regardless of the method, however, recovery from a hernia operation is usually quick. Your guy will be back on his feet within a day, and he'll be encouraged to get on with daily tasks as long as he avoids heavy lifting for three to six weeks.

Male Pain

Finally, we have a catch-all category of nonspecific aches and pains in or behind the testes. One possibility is hemorrhoids. Most cases ease over time, but a diet rich in fiber and liquids, along with not straining during bowel movements, will help. Another source of discomfort is too infrequent ejaculation (called "blue balls" around the locker room). Assuming that the obvious solution to infrequent ejaculation isn't available and do-it-himself solutions don't appeal, pulling up on an immovable object such as a car bumper (with knees bent and back straight) may ease the symptoms. For pain that doesn't have an obvious source, I have had great success referring patients to a certain physical therapist who is knowledgeable in the anatomy and disorders of the pelvic floor. There may be other physical therapists who have this same area of interest and expertise, but it may take some effort to find them.

Chances are, however, that you won't hear anything about such symptoms. Most men are inclined to suffer all but the most serious pain in silence. When he seems sullen, distant, or even grumpy, don't assume that he's angry with you. He may not be feeling well. It can take real skill to get him to admit it and describe his symptoms, but it's an important step on his road to wellness.

22

Being with Him in Sickness

My approach through most of this book has been to help you help your man prevent disease. It's easier and a lot more fun to prevent a health problem than to overcome one. Still, despite best efforts, your man can get sick, and if he does, you will most likely become his caregiver. On a practical level you will need to learn what to do. On an emotional level you also have to learn how to weather the trials of his illness, for a man who's been betrayed by his body can be a real handful.

In my experience there are three keys to success for a man facing serious illness. First, the healthier he is to begin with, and particularly if he's not overweight, the quicker he'll recover. Second, if he's motivated to recover and participates in his care, rather than just being carried along, he'll get through more easily. Last but far from least, the more involved his partner is, the sooner and more thoroughly he will heal.

Let's first talk about the stages of treatment and how you can play a role. Then we'll move on to some specific situations.

Getting Him to See a Doctor

Your biggest battle may well be convincing him to get help in the first place. Men have an unbelievable capacity for denial. I've seen men who postponed seeking treatment until they were literally on the ragged edge of life—guys who hadn't been able to urinate in three days, a man with a testicle the size of a grapefruit. Most of the time their wives made the appointment and dragged them in.

With a man deep in denial, you'll just burn out if you make an all-out appeal while his symptoms are still mild. Suggest seeing a doctor but save your real ammo for when you have a better shot at success. As he feels worse, his resolve will break down. Then you can make the big push, so save some energy.

One way to help a man face reality is to let him read about his own symptoms. Rather than tell him what you think might be wrong, hand him this book or a general reference on health and let him diagnose his own problem. Fear of the unknown keeps him from acting. The more he knows, the more likely he is to get on with it. The sooner he starts taking control of his own health, the better his chances of quick recovery.

When He Is in the Hospital

Every person entering the medical system should have an advocate backing them up, and in your man's case you're the best candidate—not because you'll have to demand the best treatment in order to get it, although you should prepared to if necessary, but because two heads (three if you count the doctor) are always better than one. Your spouse will be faced with an overwhelming amount of medical information and will have to make important decisions about treatment. Having someone at his side to help absorb and understand this information and choose treatments can be vital, particularly if he's distracted by pain and other symptoms of his illness. What is more, women typically are much more experienced with doctors and the medical system—from childbirth, for example—than men are.

With the exception of surgery and certain unusual situations, the doctor should always welcome your presence, especially if information is being conveyed or if decisions are being made. However, don't burn yourself out at your man's bedside. You're being counted on to be the alert one, so take care of yourself, too. Find out when his doctor makes rounds; you can maximize your effectiveness by being there when the doctor comes by.

Some of the hardest times will be the waiting. The hours before surgery are rough on both of you, but during surgery you'll do all the worrying. Within the limitations of staffing, you should be kept up to date about his progress and condition. In a one- or two-hour surgery this may not be necessary, but if it's longer than two hours, ask for reports.

One of the best ways to ease a man's worries before surgery is to talk to another guy who's been through the same thing. Once they've recovered, I ask my surgical patients if they'd be willing to talk to other men who are about to go through what they did. Many are happy to help out another man and can offer a man's perspective on the situation. Check with your spouse's doctor to see if this can be arranged.

Nonsurgical treatments can also pose challenges for both of you. For example, although radiation or chemotherapy may not require extensive hospitalization, they can have a big impact on both of your lives. These treatments can cause hair loss, fatigue, nausea, and other side effects. We'll talk more about cancer treatment later in this chapter.

During a lengthy stay in the hospital or confinement at home, the rest of the world can seem very far away. Encourage friends and coworkers to stop by and see him. They needn't stay long—it's often best if they don't—but a regular stream of visitors helps him reconnect with the outside world. Likewise, flowers brighten the often bland decor of a hospital room and remind him of the folks who care. Photographs of the children—or some of their artwork—can be a real boost, too.

Intimacy will be a major challenge now and during his recovery. Obviously, sex may be out of the question for a little while, but don't stop touching. If you're worried that you might hurt him, ask him if it would be okay. I'll just about guarantee a positive answer. Once again, remember that he's probably feeling very disconnected from humanity, and touching will help far more than words. When the time arrives for more than a passing caress—sooner than you may think—you'll both be more than ready.

Once He's Home Again

The day he checks out of the hospital will be momentous. It marks the beginning of his reentry into the everyday world. Even if he's had outpatient surgery, there will be relief from the waiting and worrying. From then on, although there may be times of great distress, things will be looking up. Of course his release from the medical system won't end the period during which he requires close care. Your burden will become greater once he's home.

As a rule of thumb, encourage him do a little more than you think he should—but, of course, no more than the doctor recommends. Once healing is well established, recovery requires pushing one's self back into activity. Taking those first steps won't necessarily be easy or entirely comfortable, but the longer he stays down, the harder it will be for him to get back up again. Also, the more you treat him like an invalid, the more he's likely to feel like one.

One of the most important aspects of home recovery is to establish a routine for medications. That way they get taken, and they get taken when they should. If he has powerful pain medications, don't worry too much about addiction because this is very rare. Pain medicines are there to help him get through, and he should use them as he needs them. Encourage him not to be macho and tough it out. It's much easier to nip pain in the bud than it is to knock down major pain once it's taken hold. Don't let pain get out of hand before he reaches for a pill; by then it will take bigger dosages to do the job.

Recovery is a great time to catch up on reading, so keep a big supply of books, magazines, and newspapers by the bedside. In the long run they'll be much more satisfying than television. Still, TV and radio can have their place in convalescence. They offer glimpses into the outside world that can help a guy start to feel a part of it all again. When you can, sit with him while he watches or listens, and discuss what's going on out there.

These days surgical patients do much of their recovering at home. Hospital stays have been trimmed to cut costs, so the bedroom becomes the recovery room. On the whole this works well. Most people find comfort in familiar surroundings and get better more quickly. Unfortunately, friends haven't adapted their visiting behavior to this new pattern. They may stop by faithfully while he's in the hospital but be scarce once he's arrived home. A little prodding on your part can help. The occasional hand of gin rummy or hearts with a pal will brighten your guy's day. What's more, a visit creates a good time for you to run those errands that have been stacking up or to have a little time for yourself.

Also consider arranging for regular visits from a nurse. In certain situations, for example managing incisions or catheters, insurance will pay for these visits, and you shouldn't hesitate to ask for help.

Finally, be sure that he gets outside as much as possible. Just sitting on the porch can be invigorating. Each day should contain goals and action, however small. Waiting for recovery will only extend it. Reaching for recovery will help him begin to take control of his life again.

Coming Back from Heart Problems

Recovering from a heart attack or heart surgery can be enormously difficult because most men who've had such a problem have let themselves go physically. Just recovering to the degree of health he had before the crisis won't be enough. He must become healthy enough to avoid future heart problems. It's not an easy road, but for the first time in his life he *may* have the motivation to take it.

Why "may"? Because his psychological battle can be even more difficult than his physical one. A man who's had a heart attack typically feels embarrassment over his physical failure, depression over his inadequacy as a man, and anger that his body has failed him. Depression often follows a heart attack, and you should watch for its symptoms. A few counseling sessions with a professional may be called for because depression can be serious business. Men who are depressed after a heart attack are four times as likely to die within the next six months as those who aren't. Even if he doesn't become depressed, he's likely to need a lot of encouragement and positive reinforcement from you.

Your biggest fear, and likely his as well, will be overdoing it and bringing on another heart attack. His cardiologist should provide strict guidelines for activity, and you can be certain that they will include progressively more of it. Your guy will eventually have to walk briskly for at least half an hour at least three times per week. It certainly won't hurt you to tag along.

What about more intimate activities? Once he has his doctor's clearance, sex should become a part of your lives again. You're likely to be concerned that he'll put too much stress on his heart, but research shows that's quite unlikely. Less than 1 percent of heart attacks appear to be triggered by sexual activity, and people who've had a heart attack are no more likely to suffer another one during sex than they were to have the first one then.

The reason is simple: Sex isn't as strenuous as many of us imagine. In a typical act of intercourse, a man expends about as much energy as he would climbing two flights of stairs. That may be too much early in his recovery, but most men are well enough physically within about a month of a heart attack. Don't be surprised if he's emotionally reluctant, however. His heart attack may have seriously cut into his image of himself as manly. Remember that circulatory problems also often spell erection problems, so if impotence develops, he should see his doctor. In most cases gentle coaxing and support should bring him along.

When he is ready for sex, it will help him feel more like a normal guy again and will relax him, both of which will speed his recovery. In fact, stress has been found to more than double the risk of a heart attack in the hour after it occurs, so keeping him mellow can pay dividends for his health.

Diet will also become a vital part of his move toward better health. If he wasn't ready to swear off burgers and fries before heart trouble, he should be afterward. You can refer to chapter 7 for detailed information about healthful eating. A man recovering from heart problems has to avoid saturated and partially hydrogenated fats, and cholesterol. At most his total fat intake shouldn't exceed 20 percent, and the less that's saturated or partially hydrogenated, the better. Sources of cholesterol should simply be avoided. Whether an extremely low fat diet (less than 10 percent of calories) can actually reverse heart disease remains controversial, but it appears to do no harm as long as it doesn't become a substitute for exercise and proper medical care. If he keeps the fat content of his diet low, that should also help him lose weight, which also lowers the risk of another heart attack.

Life After a Stroke

Stroke is the leading cause of long-term disability in the United States. A stroke is caused by a blocked artery or blood hemorrhage in the brain. About 550,000 Americans have strokes each year, more of them men than women. Of those, 150,000 don't survive. The other 400,000 don't fare well at all. A third have another stroke within five years. Two-thirds have some degree of impairment.

The most important way you can help your partner recover from a stroke is to see that he receives medical attention as soon as possible after symptoms begin. We reviewed those symptoms back in chapter 5, but this is so important that I'm going to repeat them here:
• Sudden weakness or numbness of one side of the face, an arm, or a leg
• Sudden dimness or loss of vision, particularly in one eye
• Loss of speech or the ability to understand speech
• Sudden severe headache without other cause
• Dizziness, unsteadiness, or falls, especially along with any of the other symptoms

Minor episodes of these symptoms—called transient ischemic attacks, or TIAs—often go unrecognized, yet they portend a more serious stroke and so should always be brought to your doctor's attention. Why is it so important to get early treatment for stroke? Clot-busting drugs developed in past few years (TPA, for example) can dramatically reduce the impact of stroke. In a study sponsored by the National Institutes of Health, the drug completely reversed the effects of stroke almost a third of the time. However, clot-busting drugs only work if they're given within the first three to six hours, and sooner is better.

Unfortunately, less than half of stroke victims get to an emergency room within three hours because they don't know the symptoms. Also, stroke victims rarely understand what's happening to them and are often incapable of getting themselves to an emergency room. They're dependent on the people around them, and that's likely to be you.

When the stroke cuts off the blood supply to part of the brain, brain cells die. This can cause paralysis on one side of the body. After a stroke, between 25 and 40 percent of people have trouble speaking, reading, writing, or understanding conversation. A speech pathologist will work with a neurologist to determine the problems and develop a rehabilitation program. Therapy may begin very soon after your loved one has a stroke because it is thought to stimulate the brain as it heals. With professional physical and speech therapy, about two-thirds of stroke victims are eventually able to return to their former activities.

Although there will be regular sessions with the speech pathologist, you and other family and friends can help a lot. Because he can't communicate well, it may not be apparent that he needs you there. He does! Converse directly with him and in an adult manner using a normal tone of voice. He may be able to hear and understand perfectly well. At the same time, don't speak rapidly and do pause frequently to allow plenty of time for him to process the words. It's also best to converse one-on-one with minimal distractions, such as other conversations or the TV. If you work together on his "homework," remember that this is truly hard work for him. He may well become agitated and angry; be prepared to accept that. It's exhausting and terribly frustrating when you can't communicate your thoughts to others.

Communication problems and feelings of isolation often lead to depression after a stroke. For some people depression may be a direct result of tissue damage in the brain. Watch for signs of depression and seek therapy or medical help if you see them.

Another common aftereffect of stroke is unpredictable emotional changes. Your man may not act like his former self. He may cry, laugh, be irritable, or be withdrawn. It may help you to know that he cannot control these emotions. You will need to learn to adjust to these uncharacteristic moods. It may help to join a support group for people who have had strokes and their families.

Managing Diabetes

Like other diseases, it is better to prevent diabetes than treat it. If your spouse would exercise five times a week, his risk of developing the most common type of diabetes would drop by 42 percent. Even one workout per week would cut that risk by 23 percent. Between 90 and 95 percent of diabetes is type 2 (also called noninsulin-dependent or adult-onset diabetes). It's becoming increasingly clear that type 2 diabetes is a lifestyle ailment.

Diabetes develops when the body has insufficient insulin (a hormone produced by the pancreas) to process sugar, raising blood sugar levels too high. There are about 700,000 Americans who produce little or no insulin and develop diabetes by their early teens (called insulin-dependent diabetes, or type 1); the other 15 million-plus diabetics make at least some insulin but became resistant to it as they grew older. Type 2 diabetes usually develops after age forty. About 90 percent of people with it are overweight. Fat cells don't respond well to insulin, causing blood sugar to rise.

Diabetes symptoms can be hard to recognize. The most obvious ones are fatigue, frequent urination, unusual thirst and hunger, weight loss, blurred vision, slow healing of sores, and tingling or loss of feeling in the hands or feet. Often, however, no obvious warning signs show up for a long time. The blood test included in a physical can help detect early signs of diabetes. A positive result should be confirmed with a fasting glucose-tolerance test. He will prepare for this test by eating a carbohydrate-rich diet for three days, then fasting overnight. He's given a concentrated sugar solution, then his blood glucose levels are monitored for three to five hours to see how he reacts.

Forty years ago all diabetics received insulin injections. Today many cases are controlled or even reversed by taking up exercise and switching to a diet low in fat and sugar, and rich in complex carbohydrates. The development of the glycemic index, a ranking of foods according to how quickly they boost blood glucose levels, has helped diabetics stabilize these levels. His doctor should be able to supply you with a glycemic index list, or you can find one on the World Wide Web.

When lifestyle changes don't control a diabetic's blood sugar levels, insulin isn't the only solution. Three oral medications may help. Sulfonylureas stimulate the pancreas to produce more insulin. Because their use often leads to weight gain, however, they're best for those without a weight problem. Metformin reduces the amount of sugar released by the liver, a better approach for obese diabetics. In rare instances (particularly during serious illness), however, it can lead to a dangerous condition in which sugar is incompletely metabolized. If your spouse takes Metformin and is admitted to the hospital, be sure the doctors know he's taking it. Finally, there's acarbose, which slows the breakdown of carbohydrates into sugar. Side effects with acarbose are generally limited to indigestion.

When exercise, weight loss, and combinations of the oral medications aren't sufficient, insulin injections may be in order. They are still the most effective way to keep blood sugar levels under control, and they work especially well when combined with a healthier lifestyle.

If your man has diabetes, it is vital that he control it. If he doesn't, the health consequences will be great. Each year 24,000 diabetics become blind, 56,000 develop kidney failure, 78,000 die from heart disease or stroke, and 54,000 have a leg amputated. After twenty-five years of poorly controlled diabetes, more than half of people will show some signs of nerve damage (diabetic neuropathy). In men that often means impotence; one-third of diabetic men can't get or sustain an erection. He doesn't have to end up there. Help him help himself to better health.

Surviving Cancer

Of all the life-threatening diseases discussed in this chapter, cancer is undoubtedly the most frightening to both a man and his partner. If heart disease, stroke, and diabetes spell betrayal of a man by his body, cancer amounts to an invasion. He may feel that a battle is going on inside his body.

To keep such negative attitudes in check, remind him (and yourself) that most cancers are quite survivable. Over 40 percent of people diagnosed with cancer are alive five years later, including people with lung cancer, which is the second most common and one of the least survivable cancers. The American Cancer Society estimates that 98,300 men were diagnosed with lung cancer in 1997, and 94,400 died of it; 334,500 were diagnosed with prostate cancer, but only 41,800 died of it. For most forms of cancer the odds that you have a number of happy years together ahead of you are much better than you both may imagine.

You can increase those odds and make the intervening years more pleasant by taking an active role in helping him recover from cancer. Long term, many of the lifestyle changes are the same ones used to avoid cancer in the first place: diet and exercise.

There are many ways you can help make his cancer treatments—whether they be surgery, radiation, or chemotherapy—more comfortable and effective. I suggest you pick up a copy of *The Cancer Recovery Eating Plan* by Daniel W. Nixon, M.D., which covers not only diet but other approaches. As Dr. Nixon points out, individual responses to treatment are extremely variable, so choose the solution that best fits your man's situation.

Fatigue is a common—and commonly ignored—side effect of any treatment for cancer. Nearly 80 percent of patients experience it, and nearly two-thirds say it affects everyday life more than pain. Sadly, less than a third mention it to their doctor, and most doctors consider it less important to treat than pain. Too many people simply suffer through it. Fatigue can be a direct result of anemia from chemotherapy, it may be caused by poor nutrition, or it can stem from psychological factors. All these causes can be treated, reducing if not eliminating fatigue. If your man shows signs of fatigue, be sure that he brings it to the attention of his doctor.

Learn when he's likely to be most energetic—is he a morning person or a night owl?—and schedule activities for those times. Mild exercise when he's feeling chipper will boost his energy level. Also make room for rest periods. One a day may do the job, or it may take four or five. These should be periods of true relaxation, but try to save sleeping for the night to avoid nighttime insomnia.

Nutritionally he may benefit from eating small amounts every couple of hours rather than three meals four or five hours apart. Be prepared for his tastes in food to make a total flip-flop. During cancer recovery his usual favorites may be utterly unappealing. Ask what tastes good and experiment.

Nausea may accompany chemotherapy and sometimes radiation. If your guy experiences nausea during treatment, and especially if he vomits, talk to his doctor about an antinausea medication. Ondansetron will solve the problem most of the time.

You can also lessen nausea with eating strategies. He may do better if he eats before a treatment session or if he has an empty stomach. It helps to write these events down in a notebook so you can keep track of what's working and what's not. Many people do well by reverting to foods that were comforting when they were young, whether it's chicken soup or ginger ale. Concentrate on liquids, especially if he's vomiting or has diarrhea. He shouldn't be choosing diet drinks because he can use the sugar at this point.

Tips That May Help Control Nausea

- Offer lots of liquids but not at mealtimes.
- Have him eat slowly small amounts of carbohydrate—plain crackers, for example—every thirty to sixty minutes.
- When he's nauseated, salty foods may work better than sweet ones.
- Feed him a small amount of carbohydrate as soon as he wakes up in the morning. (It worked for morning sickness, didn't it?)
- If he becomes nauseous at a particular time or after a particular event, avoid having a favorite food around then. You don't want them to become associated in his mind.
- Try to avoid cooking odors in the house. They may set things off.
- Have him sit up or lie propped up for at least two hours after eating.
- A lemon or peppermint candy or even chewing gum may help when he's being given chemotherapy.
- Suggest he brush his teeth or rinse his mouth out frequently. It may lessen nausea and will help avoid tooth decay, a common problem during chemotherapy.
- A cool, damp towel on the back of his neck may help.
- Open a window or take him for a walk in the fresh air.

Whether he's nauseous or just lacks appetite, getting adequate nutrition can be a real problem for a man undergoing cancer treatment. The trick is to concentrate calories and protein without adding fat. Powdered milk will be one of your most important tools for getting protein into him. You can add it to skim milk to make it seem like whole milk; mix it into low-fat yogurt (along with fruit); supplement casseroles, hot cereals, and breads with a few tablespoons; or even stir some into a milk shake. Dried fruits can be an important caloric ally since they combine well with a variety of dishes. And don't hesitate to add sugar to recipes as long as the sweetness doesn't trigger nausea. You might even consider some of those health food store protein shake mixes if his doctor approves. Finally, his diet is likely to concentrate on a few foods, so his nutritional needs may not be fully met. Consider giving him a multivitamin to add important vitamins and minerals.

Dry mouth commonly accompanies radiation therapy and may not disappear once the treatment is over. Antinausea drugs can also cause it. The first line of treatment is lots of water. He will find soft, damp, cool, or lukewarm foods easier to chew and swallow. Sucking on ice chips or sugar-free candies or chewing sugar-free gum may help. (Although sugar is useful once it reaches the digestive tract, dry mouth increases the risk of tooth decay. Get the sugar down quickly and have him brush or rinse his mouth out.)

Changes in bowel habits often happen during cancer treatments, but it's important to report any significant changes to his doctor. Constipation may be triggered by some anticancer drugs or by pain medications. Encourage him to head off the problem by drinking lots of liquids, eating plenty of fiber-containing foods, and getting as much exercise as possible. Diarrhea, on the other hand, can be caused by surgery, radiation, chemotherapy, antibiotics, or even antinausea medicines. Once again, liquids are very important, but avoid those that contain caffeine. You might try discontinuing milk products to see if the treatments have caused him to become intolerant of lactose (a dairy sugar). Perhaps your best bet, short of Kaopectate, is to feed him the BRAT diet, a technique hospitals have used for years. The combination of bananas, rice, applesauce, and toast (all plain) has a profoundly soothing effect on the intestines.

Get Help for Yourself, Too

Nursing a man back to health can be exhausting—and even more so when the caregiver is also trying to maintain a household, take care of children or her parents, keep a job, or cope with her own health problems. This is no time to tough it out on your own. This is what parents, friends, employers, and even in-laws are for. Let someone else keep the house standing and the kids fed. Be clear with your work supervisor that you need this time. Give yourself the space you need to concentrate on taking care of him—and yourself, too.

Don't underestimate the psychological strain. Not only has the number one person in your life gone through a horrible time, but the foundations of your life have been threatened. Talk about your feelings with friends and family. You need both logistical and mental support during this time. If you take good care of yourself, you can take good care of him, and life will turn the right corner much quicker. If the man you love has a health problem that will affect his life and yours for years to come, it's especially important that you think of your own needs.

Keeping Your Relationship Strong

When your man is going through recovery or is facing long-term illness, your relationship will change. You will have to learn to be a caregiver, and he will have to learn to be a care receiver. Here are some suggestions that can help you cope with the changed dynamics.

• **Treat him with respect.** You can nurture his self-esteem by including him in daily plans, even if the decisions seem trivial to you. Include him when deciding what to have for lunch or what you'll watch on TV. It will also bolster his pride to get cleaned up and dressed every day.

• **Communicate with each other.** There's never been a more important time to be honest and open. Don't assume you know his needs and emotions, and make sure to tell him yours.

• **Give yourself a break.** Ask a friend or relative, or hire a caregiver or visiting nurse, to relieve you for a couple of hours a few times a week. If your partner has a long-term disability, you may want to explore adult daycare options.

• **Take care of you.** Keep up with your hobbies and interests, and stay connected to current events and to your friends. Ask your doctor, hospital, or patient organization about a support group for caregivers. If you don't take care of yourself, you're both going to be in trouble.

Afterword

These are complicated and often difficult times for men and women. It's easy to lose sight of what really matters in your life. The time to love a child or make love with your spouse competes with jobs, social obligations, bills to be paid, and traffic jams.

I'm only a doctor, just one man, and I can't tell you and your partner how to manage those demands. I can tell both of you, though, that peak health—the kind we get from exercise, a careful diet, and preventive medicine—will give you the best possible chance of successfully meeting all your obligations and desires.

Over the past twenty-two chapters we've covered a lot of pain and not a little potential joy. At least as important, I've also described a lot of men and their predicaments. Perhaps none of those men turned out to be just like yours, but I hope that some of the lessons my patients and their partners have learned prove helpful to you and yours. It's my most devout wish that it be so.

Share Sheets

The following are briefing papers and checklists you can copy and pass along to your partner.

Eating Better on the Job or on the Road

- **Breakfast in a hotel:** Steer clear of the buffet. Instead, order some juice, cereal with skim milk or low-fat yogurt, fresh fruit, and a bagel or dry toast. It will cost less, you'll be just as full, and you'll save hundreds of calories.
- **Donuts in the office:** Sure, they're tempting, but wouldn't you rather save all those calories for something that lasts longer and is more satisfying?
- **The fast-food lunch:** It's not easy eating well from the take-out window, but it can be done. Order the broiled chicken sandwich with no sauce. Add mustard and ketchup to suit. Unsweetened ice tea is a good drink choice, but if you really have the urge, order a milk shake. Most have little milk in them and actually are fairly low in fat. Need I say no french fries? Some places have baked potatoes or salad choices.
- **Mid-afternoon snack:** What, this isn't a normal work routine? Make it one. Carry a piece of fruit or no-fat fig bars for an afternoon boost. Hard-boiled eggs are also good—only the white if you have trouble with cholesterol. The snack will keep you going when others are slowing, and you won't be starved come dinnertime.
- **Dinner:** Restaurants want to make you happy by making you full of fatty calories. Don't let them do it! Choose chicken or fish dishes over beef, and whatever you order, ask for the sauce on the side. That goes for salad dressing as well. A baked potato is a great choice as long as you can skip the butter or sour cream. Salsa is a wonderful substitute. Chinese food is a good choice, but stick with the lighter sauces—on the side—and vegetable, tofu, or shrimp dishes. If you minimize sauces and learn to eat bread sans the butter, you'll probably be able to have dessert—sorbet, at least.

Getting Ready for Your Checkup

- **Records:** If you're changing doctors, ask the old office to send over your records. (This can take a couple of weeks.)
- **Test prep:** Find out if there is anything you should avoid before having a test (eating, having sex, etc.). Find out if you can have any blood test in advance since the analysis takes a few days. That way the doctor can explain the results in person.
- **Make lists:** Write down things to tell the doctor and questions you'd like answered. Doctor visits are famous for causing amnesia.
- **Complaints:** Had a particular ache or pain lately? Indigestion? Dizziness? Think about when it happened, what you were doing at the time, how it felt, and what makes it feel better so that you can explain the problem clearly.
- **Family history:** You should come prepared with a list of health problems that have affected your brothers, father, and grandfather. Heart disease, alcoholism, diabetes? Knowing you're at risk can help you avoid them.
- **Medications:** Bring a list of your meds—not only prescription drugs but over-the-counter ones, too. Do you use a lot of antacids, sleeping pills, or even aspirin? Herbal remedies? Vitamins? Each will tell the doctor something about your condition.
- **Goals:** What would you like to improve about your health? Do you really want to quit smoking, cut back on drinking, or build some endurance? If the doctor can't help directly, he knows where you can find help.
- **Questions:** Have you been wondering about the latest advice on eating eggs? Would you like to know if that glass of wine each day will hurt you? You'll never remember to ask if you don't write those questions down.

A Dozen Questions to Ask Your Relatives

Until you get used to the idea, it's not easy interviewing your relatives about health. Use this list of questions to start, and adapt them as you gain experience. If possible, the best person to interview first may be your mother.

1. How are you feeling today? Do you have any health troubles? (If no, go to 5.)

2. Are you seeing a doctor about it or are you taking a medication?

3. How long have you had this problem?

4. Did any of your parents or brothers and sisters have this problem? If so, which ones?

5. How is Dad's/Mom's health? Does he/she have any troublesome health problems? (If no, go to 9.)

6. Does he/she see a doctor about it or take a medication?

7. How long has he/she had this problem?

8. Do you know if any of his/her parents or brothers and sisters had this problem?

9. Do you know what your father/grandfather/great-grandfather died from? Did he have other problems that contributed to his decline? (A man with prostate cancer may die from pneumonia.)

10. Do you know of any problems such as depression or alcoholism among your relatives? (If you're talking with a sensitive relative, ask whether the person liked a drink or two.)

11. Do you know of anyone in our family line who has had diabetes, heart disease, or prostate, colon, or testicular cancer?

12. Can you think of anything else about our relatives' health that might be of interest?

Eventually you should fill in the following sheet for as many blood relatives as you can, particularly your father, grandfathers, and any brothers.

Name
Relation
Year of birth
Year of death
Cause of death
Disorders
    Heart attack
    High blood pressure
    High cholesterol
    Chest pain (angina)
    Coronary bypass surgery
    Heart disease
    Stroke
    Lung cancer
    Colon cancer
    Other cancer (type?)
    Diabetes
    Allergies (including medications)
    Depression or other psychological conditions
    Alcoholism
Lifestyle
    Overweight?
    Smoked?
    Drinker? (heavy, moderate, or not)
Medications

Pain and Gain

Men are renowned for saying "I don't want to talk about it" when it comes to their health, but much of the time we're really saying "I don't know *how* to talk about it." We don't spend a lot of time thinking about how to describe our pain because we're trying to forget it. But a man who can really spell out his pain is a man who can help his doctor figure out how to make it stop. Here are some descriptions to help you start to develop a vocabulary for pain and other health problems.

Ache: Subtly different from a dull pain, aches tend to be there when we sit or lie down too long. That knee that had a dull pain after the tennis game may ache when you get up the next morning.

Burning pain: Maybe this one happens above your stomach after a particularly heavy meal, or perhaps it happens sometimes when you wait too long to urinate.

Dull pain: The pain we try to convince ourselves isn't there. Maybe you feel it in a knee for only a few hours after a tennis game. Trouble is, it's been lasting longer and longer.

Grabbing pain: The kind that can double you over, this one's hard to ignore.

Sharp pain: Does the stitch in your side nearly double you over? Is that calf cramp causing you to wince? That's a sharp pain.

Spasms: From an uncontrollable muscle in the abdomen to a clamped-down bladder, a spasm is obvious when it's happening but easy to forget when it passes.

Throbbing pain: Miss a nail with a hammer and substitute your thumb— that's throbbing pain. Setting a piece of furniture down on a toe could rightly be described that way.

Symptoms That Should Send You to the Doctor

These general symptoms don't necessarily mean that you're on the brink of disaster, but they occur often enough with serious diseases that it's always worth checking them out. With the really bad news ruled out, you can relax.

- Weight loss of ten pounds or more for no apparent reason
- Regular or constant thirst for no apparent reason
- Frequent need to urinate despite not drinking excessively
- Fatigue without apparent reason
- A sore on the skin or in the mouth that doesn't heal
- A lump that appears under the skin
- Recurrent headache accompanied by vomiting
- Headache that persists for several hours despite taking medication
- Sudden severe headache without other cause
- Pain or tightness in the chest, especially during exertion
- Chest pain that radiates to your neck, jaws, or down your back
- Pain in your jaws, arms, or back
- Unusual shortness of breath
- Dizziness, fainting, sweating, nausea, or weakness
- Indigestion that doesn't respond to antacids
- Erection problems
- Sudden weakness or numbness of one side of the face and an arm or leg
- Sudden dimness or loss of vision, particularly in one eye
- Loss of speech or the ability to understand speech
- Difficulty swallowing
- Persistent cough, hoarseness, or loss of voice
- Coughing up blood
- A change in bowel habits or stool appearance
- Pink urine
- Painful or difficult urination
- A lump in a testicle
- Unusual mood swings, including anxiety, depression, or distraction
- Changes in sleep patterns

American Urological Association's Benign Prostatic Hyperplasia (BPH) Symptom Checklist

Do you feel as if you're spending half of your life in the bathroom these days and not seeing much result for all the effort? You may have an enlarged prostate, especially if you're over fifty. Review the questions below and answer them as accurately as you can. The results will help you and your urologist determine whether you should have some tests, and perhaps treatment, to set things right. Even if your score is on the low side, don't hesitate to make that doctor visit. Other easily curable problems can cause urinary troubles. Above all, don't stay away from the clinic because you're afraid a diagnosis will mean surgery. These days, medication can usually do the job.

Circle one answer for each question. Then add up your scores.

1. Over the past month, how often have you had a sensation of not emptying your bladder completely after you finished urinating?
Never (score 0)
Less than 1 time in 5 (score 1)
Less than half the time (2)
About half the time (3)
More than half the time (4)
Almost always (5)

2. Over the past month, how often have you had to urinate again less than two hours after you finished urinating?
Never (score 0)
Less than 1 time in 5 (score 1)
Less than half the time (2)
About half the time (3)
More than half the time (4)
Almost always (5)

3. Over the past month, how often have you found that you stopped and started again several times when you urinated?
Never (score 0)
Less than 1 time in 5 (score 1)
Less than half the time (2)
About half the time (3)
More than half the time (4)
Almost always (5)

4. Over the past month, how often have you found it difficult to postpone urination?
Never (score 0)
Less than 1 time in 5 (score 1)
Less than half the time (2)
About half the time (3)
More than half the time (4)
Almost always (5)

5. Over the past month, how often have you had a weak urinary stream?
Never (score 0)
Less than 1 time in 5 (score 1)
Less than half the time (2)
About half the time (3)
More than half the time (4)
Almost always (5)

6. Over the past month, how often have you had to push or strain to begin urination?
Never (score 0)
Less than 1 time in 5 (score 1)
Less than half the time (2)
About half the time (3)
More than half the time (4)
Almost always (5)

7. Over the past month, how many times did you most typically get up to urinate from the time you went to bed at night until the time you got up in the morning?

None (score 0)

1 time (1)

2 times (2)

3 times (3)

4 times (4)

5 times (5)

Add up the numbers. Symptoms are classified as mild (1–9), moderate (10–19), or severe (20–35). Generally, no treatment is needed for mild symptoms; moderate symptoms may need treatment; and severe symptoms almost always require treatment.

Take this quiz with you to a urologist. He'll be impressed at how well you've done your homework, and you'll be well on your way to finding the solution that works for you.

Skin Self-Exam

Skin cancer is the most common malignant tumor. By keeping watch over your skin, you can discover a problem before it becomes serious. Look at moles and spots everywhere, not just the parts exposed to the sun. You and your partner could check each other out. This opens up interesting possibilities, doesn't it? Look for:

Asymmetrical shape: Any mole or spot on the skin that doesn't have a round shape is worth showing to a doctor.

Borders: Irregular borders identify a mole or spot that's worth taking a closer look at.

Color: Changes across the surface of the mole or spot should bring it to your attention and that of a doctor.

Diameter: If it's larger than a standard pencil eraser, the mole or spot ought to be examined by a professional.

Remember: A, B, C, D.

Breast Self-Exam

Although breast cancer occurs in only about 1 out of every 100,000 men, it does happen. Early diagnosis gives the best hope for a complete cure. Breast self-exam in men differs only slightly from that in women. It's easy to do, but you might consider asking her to show you since she's probably been doing these every month for years. Get in the habit of doing this once a month—the first day of the month is easy to remember.

1. Stand in front of a mirror and look for any irregularities, puckering, or changes in shape (compare the two sides). Get a good idea of what you normally look like so you have a baseline.

2. With the pads of the fingers of your left hand, press gently in decreasing circles, from the outside in, feeling for lumps. (You're most likely to find one near the nipple.)

3. Using the same technique, examine the side of your chest and up toward the armpit.

4. Repeat the procedure using the right hand for the left side.

5. Keep track of any lumps and look for changes over time. If you feel a lump or thickening, see your doctor.

Testicular Self-Exam

To find testicular cancer when it's still curable, examine your testes at least once a month. The best time is in the shower when your scrotum is relaxed.

1. Grasp each testicle between your thumb and first two fingers, with your thumb behind.
2. Gently run your fingers around the circumference of each testicle feeling for lumps or hard places.
3. The testicle should feel like a small hard-boiled egg without its shell.
4. In the back, where your thumb is, you may find a lump called the epididymis; the rest of the surface should be smooth and pliable.
5. Get used to what your testes feel like and report any change to your doctor.

Cancer Symptoms

1. Change in bowel or bladder habits
- thinner stool
- different color of urine or stool
- different frequency
2. A sore that doesn't heal
3. Unusual bleeding or discharge
- in the ejaculate
- in the stool
- in the urine
- coughing up blood
4. A lump or thickening
- in a testicle
- under the arm
- in a breast
5. Indigestion or difficulty swallowing
6. Obvious change in a wart or mole
7. Nagging cough or hoarseness

Resources

Hotlines

Agency for Health Care Policy Research	(800) 358-9295
AIDS Hotline	(800) 342-2437
American Academy of Family Physicians	(800) 274-2237
American Association of Sex Educators, Counselors, and Therapists	(312) 644-0828
American Cancer Society	(800) 227-2345
American Council on Alcoholism	(800) 527-5344
American Council on Exercise	(800) 529-8227
American Diabetes Association	(800) 232-3472
American Dietetic Association	(800) 366-1655
American Foundation for Urological Diseases	(800) 242-2383
American Heart Association	(214) 706-1179
American Institute of Preventive Medicine	(800) 345-2476
Cancer Information Service (NIH)	(800) 422-6237
Center for Disease Control	(404) 639-3311
Center for Science in the Public Interest	(202) 332-9110
Environmental Protection Agency	(800) 535-0202
Food and Nutrition Information Center	(301) 504-5719
Help for Incontinent People	(800) 252-3337
Herpes Hotline	(919) 361-8488
HPV (Condyloma) Support Program	(919) 361-8400
Impotence Institute of America	(800) 669-1603
Library of Medicine	(301) 496-4000
Medicare Hotline	(800) 638-6833
Men's Health Network	(202) 543-6461
National Center for Health Statistics	(301) 436-8500
National Council on Alcoholism and Drug Dependency	(800) 622-2255
National Council on Patient Information Education	(202) 347-6711
National Drug Information and Referral	(800) 662-4357
National Health Information Center	(800) 336-4797

National Headache Foundation............................ (800) 843-2256
National Injury Information............................... (301) 504-0424
National Institute of Health.............................. (301) 496-4000
National Institute of Health (Nutrition)................. (301) 496-9281
National Institute of Mental Health..................... (301) 443-4513
National Men's Resource Center.......................... (415) 453-2839
National Pesticide Telecommunication................... (800) 858-7378
National Radon Hotline................................... (800) 767-7236
Office on Smoking and Health............................ (404) 488-5701
People's Medical Society................................. (800) 624-8773
President's Council on Physical Fitness and Sports...... (202) 690-9000
Sexually Transmitted Disease Hotline.................... (800) 227-8922
Skin Cancer Society....................................... (212) 725-5176
U.S. Consumer Product Safety............................ (800) 638-2772
U.S. Government Occupational Safety and Health
    Administration... (800) 356-4674
Us Too Hotline.. (800) 828-7866

On the Web

The World Wide Web can be a great source of health information. Your guy may well find surfing the Internet an easy and enjoyable way to learn about his health as well as specific conditions. Since anyone can send out health information over the Internet, though, some sites are full of bunk. Look for sites sponsored by major health organizations and institutions, and associated with accredited physicians. The following sites are good starting places. Each includes links to other sites.

American Medical Association................... http://www.ama-assn.org
American Cancer Society......................... http://www.cancer.org
Male Health Center..................... http://www.malehealthcenter.com
Mayo Health Center's Oasis.................. http://www.mayohealth.org
American Foundation for Urologic Disease.......... http://www.afud.org
American Urological Association................... http://www.auanet.org
CancerNet...................... http://www.arc.com/cancernet/cancernet
CNN Interactive Health Page... http://www.cnn.com/health/index.html
Food and Drug Administration........................ http://www.fda.gov
The Prostate Foundation......................... http://www.prostate.org
Prostate Pointers.. http://www.rattler.cameron.edu/prostate/prostate.html

Bibliography

Ackerman, Robert, and Susan Pickering. *Before It's Too Late: Helping Women in Abusive or Controlling Relationships*. New York: W.H. Freeman, 1998.

Arnot, Robert, M.D. *The Best Medicine: How to Choose the Top Doctors, the Top Hospitals, and the Top Treatments*. Reading, MA: Addison-Wesley Publishing, 1992.

Benson, Herbert, M.D. (with Marg Stack). *Timeless Healing: The Power and Biology Belief*. New York: Fireside (Simon and Schuster), 1997.

Boston Women's Health Book Collective. *The New Our Bodies, Ourselves: A Book by and for Women*. New York: Touchstone (Simon and Schuster), 1992.

Butler, Robert, M.D., and Myrna Lewis, M.S.W. *Love and Sex After 60*. New York: Ballantine Books, 1993.

Crute, Sheree, ed. *Health and Healing for African-Americans: Straight Talk and Tips from More Than 150 Black Doctors on Our Top Health Concerns*. Emmaus, PA: Rodale Press, 1997.

Diamond, Jed. *Male Menopause*. Naperville, IL: Sourcebooks, 1997.

Farrell, Warren, Ph.D. *The Myth of Male Power: Why Men Are the Disposable Sex*. New York: Simon and Schuster, 1993.

Fisher, Stephen. *Colon Cancer and the Polyps Connection*. Tucson, AZ: Fisher Books, 1995.

Fried, Stephen. *Bitter Pills: Inside the Hazardous World of Legal Drugs*. New York: Bantam Books: 1998.

Gilbaugh, James, Jr., M.D. *A Doctor's Guide to Men's Private Parts*. New York: Crown Publishers, 1988.

Goldberg, Kenneth, M.D. *How Men Can Live as Long as Women*. Fort Worth, TX: Summit, 1994.

Goldman, Robert, M.D., and Robert Klatz, M.D. *Stopping the Clock: Dramatic Breakthroughs in Anti-Aging and Age Reversal Techniques*. New York: Bantam Books, 1997.

Ingram, Cass, M.D. (with Judy Gray, M.S.). *Eat Right to Live Long*. Hiawatha: Literary Visions, 1989.

Jacobowitz, Ruth. *150 Most-Asked Questions About Midlife Sex, Love, and Intimacy that Women and Their Partners Really Want to Know*. New York: William Morrow and Co., 1996.

Kaltenbach, Don (with Tim Richards). *Prostate Cancer: A Survivor's Guide*. New Port Richey, FL: Seneca House Press, 1995.

Korsch, Barbara, M.D., and Caroline Harding. *The Intelligent Patient's Guide to the Doctor-Patient Relationship: Learning How to Talk so Your Doctor Will Listen*. New York: Oxford University Press, 1997.

Lamm, Steven, M.D., and Gerald Secor Couzens. *The Virility Solution*. New York: Simon and Schuster, 1998.

Lewis, James, Jr. *How I Survived Prostate Cancer . . . and So Can You*. Westbury, NY: Health Education Literary Publisher, 1994.

Marks, Sheldon, M.D. *Prostate and Cancer: A Family Guide to Diagnosis, Treatment, and Survival*. Tucson, AZ: Fisher Books, 1995.

McGrath, Ellen, Ph.D. *When Feeling Bad Is Good*. New York: Bantam Books, 1994.

Men's Fitness Magazine with Kevin Cobb. *Complete Guide to Health and Well-Being*. New York: HarperPerennial, 1996.

Micheli, Lyle, M.D. *The Healthy Runner's Handbook*. Champaign, IL: Human Kinetics Publishers, 1996.

Micheli, Lyle, M.D. (with Mark Jenkins). *The Sports Medicine Bible: Prevent, Detect, and Treat Your Sports Injuries Through the Latest Medical Techniques*. New York: John Boswell Associates (HarperCollins), 1995.

Morgentaler, Abraham, M.D. *The Male Body: A Physician's Guide to What Every Man Should Know About His Sexual Health*. New York: Fireside Books (Simon and Schuster), 1993.

Moyers, Bill. *Healing and the Mind*. New York: Doubleday, 1993.

Nixon, Daniel W. *The Cancer Recovery Eating Plan*. New York: Times Books, 1996.

Oesterling, Joseph, M.D. *The ABCs of Prostate Cancer: The Book That Could Save Your Life*. Lanham, MD: Madison Books, 1997.

Ornish, Dean, M.D. *Dr. Dean Ornish's Program for Reversing Heart Disease*. New York: Random House, 1990.

———. *Eat More, Weigh Less: Dr. Dean Ornish's Life Choice Program for Losing Weight Safely While Eating Abundantly.* New York: HarperCollins, 1993.

———. *Love and Survival: The Scientific Basis for the Healing Power of Intimacy.* New York: HarperCollins, 1997.

Prochaska, James, Ph.D., John Norcross, Ph.D., and Carlo Diclemente, Ph.D. *Changing for Good.* New York: Avon, 1994.

Renshaw, Domeena, M.D. (with Pam Brick). *Seven Weeks to Better Sex.* New York: American Medical Association/Random House, 1995.

Rowe, John, M.D., and Robert Kahn, Ph.D. *Successful Aging.* New York: Pantheon Books, 1998.

Sapolsky, Robert M. *Why Zebras Don't Get Ulcers.* Deerfield, FL: Health Communications, 1995.

Sheehy, Gail. "Male Menopause: The Unspeakable Passage," *Vanity Fair,* April 1993.

———. *New Passages: Mapping Your Life Across Time.* New York: Random House, 1995.

———. *Understanding Men's Passages: Discovering the New Map of Men's Lives.* New York: Random House, 1998.

Wallerstein, Judith S., et al. *The Good Marriage: How and Why Love Lasts.* New York: Warner Books, 1996.

Zilbergeld, Bernie, Ph.D. *The New Male Sexuality.* New York: Bantam Books, 1992.

Index

accidents, 15, 16, 18, 20, 99, 100, 111-114, 159
Adipex-P, 106
adrenaline, 121, 157, 160
aggression, 21-23, 25, 26, 111
aging, 71, 72, 84, 104, 106, 118, 144, 184, 186, 209-215, 219
   see also older men
AIDS, 18, 175, 176-177, 210
alcohol, 15, 25, 36, 95, 114, 158, 159, 170, 184
   health effects of, 20, 58, 104, 108, 198, 239, 245
alcoholism, 54, 104, 114-115, 130, 135, 159
alpha-andrenergic blockers (alpha blockers), 236-237
Alzheimer's disease, 83, 114, 125
Anafranil, 172
angina, 54, 61-62, 275
antibiotics, 178, 181, 182, 200, 204, 224, 240-241, 247, 249, 264
antidepressants, 132-133, 172
antioxidants, 82, 222
appearance, 36, 71, 72, 75-76, 92, 115, 118
arrhythmia, 59
arteries, 34-35, 49, 62, 83, 115, 142-144, 157-158

back problems, 73, 159
balanitis, 250
balloon dilation, 238
basal cell carcinoma, 57
benign prostatic hyperplasia (BPH), *see* prostate enlargement
beta-carotene, 82, 83
biofeedback, 172
biopsy, 224-225, 228, 229, 241
bipolar disorder, 131
birth control, 20, 185-195
   see also specific methods
bladder, 139-140, 234, 238, 245-246
blood pressure check, 14, 43-44, 59-60, 159
   see also high blood pressure

blood tests, 42, 48-50, 159, 179, 211, 212, 213, 225, 260, 271
body-mass index (BMI), 89, 90
brachytherapy, 230
breakfast, 93, 270
breast cancer, 18, 19, 52, 54, 57-58, 83, 211, 212, 280

caffeine, 60, 104-105, 106, 198, 239, 264
calcium, 82, 143
calories, 91-92, 93, 95, 104, 263
cancer, 15, 17-19, 53-54, 122, 178, 201, 211, 212, 225, 261-264
   death rates from, 80, 221, 222, 248, 261
   dietary factors in, 53, 80-81, 82, 83-84, 221-222
   early detection of, 51, 53, 55, 58, 220, 248
   racial and ethnic factors in, 118, 221, 223
   seven warning signs of, 61, 282
   see also specific cancers
candidiasis, 177
carbohydrates, 79, 84, 104, 260, 263
carcinoma, 57
Cardura, 236
carotenoids, 82, 83
cataracts, 64, 82
Caverject, 166
cervical cancer, 178-179, 201
cervical cap, 184, 186, 189
chancroid, 177
change, *see* lifestyle change
checkup, *see* physical exam
chemotherapy, 248, 255, 262-263, 264
chest pain, *see* angina
chicken, 80, 82, 85, 88, 94-95, 97, 270
childbirth, 207, 254
Chinese food, 80, 86, 96, 270
chlamydia, 175, 177, 179, 200, 247
cholesterol, 14, 49-50, 54, 55, 63, 80, 82, 83, 89, 92, 122, 159, 258, 270
chronic obstructive lung disease, 18
chronotherapy, 100-101

circadian rhythm, 99-101, 109, 210-211
circumcision, 145-146, 177, 250
colonoscopy, 47
colorectal cancer, 14, 18, 46, 47, 52, 53-54, 81, 83
condoms, 17, 20, 170, 177, 179, 180, 181, 182-187
condoms, female, 182, 185, 188-189
condyloma, 178-179
conformal therapy, 230
constipation, 73, 81, 264
consultation, medical, 44-45, 113-114, 132, 158, 199, 224, 232
continuous positive airway pressure (CPAP), 108
control, need for, 23, 32, 122-125, 129-130, 133, 134
conversation, 33-34, 36, 52-53, 65, 70, 123, 256, 259, 264
   in marriage, 150, 152, 153, 171, 205, 265
cooking, 31, 79, 85-87, 93-97
cortisol, 122
counseling, 133, 159, 169, 170-171, 199
crash diets, 90-91
cryotherapy, 232
cumulative trauma syndrome (CTS), 73
cystoscopy, 235

dairy products, 80, 82, 84, 245
death, 2, 17-19, 52, 111-112, 115, 130
death rate, 2, 26, 69, 111-112, 113, 114, 119, 129, 176, 221, 222
   for cancer, 80, 221, 222, 248, 261
dehydroepiandrosterone (DHEA), 210, 211
denial, 1-5, 13, 17, 19, 21, 38, 52, 61, 64, 114-115, 152-153, 209, 234, 253-254
   of emotions, 25, 129, 131, 135-136, of fallibility, 23, 32, 122-123, 150
   of pain, 1-2, 25, 62, 129, 252
dental care, 14, 36, 45, 58, 108, 117, 263, 264
depression, 1, 35, 54, 63-64, 72, 110, 116, 122, 129-133, 199, 212, 220, 275
   illness-related, 19, 132, 257, 259
diabetes, 18, 48, 49, 50, 54, 63, 69, 75, 82, 89, 121, 122, 177, 260-261
   impotence caused by, 20, 61, 62, 158, 159, 161
diagnostic tests, 40, 42, 46-50, 204-205, 225-226, 234, 240, 271
   see also specific tests
diaphragm, 182, 184, 186, 189
diarrhea, 264

diet, 4, 7, 15, 17, 35, 36, 79-88, 91, 198, 209, 239, 244-245, 252, 260-264, 267
   away from home, 86, 95-97, 270
   cancer risk affected by, 15, 53, 80-84, 221-222, 229, 261
   change of, 31, 41, 62, 85-88, 93-97, 257-258, 260
   for high blood pressure, 41, 43-44, 82
dietary supplements, 83, 84, 210, 222, 229, 263
diethylstilbestrol (DES), 200-201, 231
digital rectal exam (DRE), 14, 46, 49, 53, 213, 222-223, 224, 226, 229, 234, 240
diverticulitis, 81
dizziness, 62, 63, 258, 275
doctor, choice of, 38-41, 156, 167, 193, 206, 235
driving, 15, 36, 99, 100, 111-113
drug abuse, 15, 36, 54, 114, 130, 184
drugs, see medication
dynamic infusion cavernosometry and cavernosography (DICC), 160
dysthmia, 131

EDEX, 166
ejaculation, 49, 141, 142, 152, 168, 193, 194, 201-204, 214, 223, 238
   health benefits of, 147, 239, 252
   premature, 145, 156, 169-173, 187
   retrograde, 140, 238
electrocardiogram (EKG), 47-48
emotions, expression of, 23, 32, 122-123, 129, 131-136, 150, 265
emphysema, 48, 54, 55
epididymitis, 247
erectile dysfunction (ED), 155-169
erection, 60-61, 142-143, 146, 151, 160, 193
erection injections, 160, 166-167
exercise, 4, 7, 41, 43-44, 48, 59, 60, 62, 69-78, 116, 154, 267
   aerobic, 36, 72, 73-74, 75, 76, 92, 123
   age and, 35, 69, 71-72, 76, 209
   depression reduced by, 72, 133
   goals for, 69-70, 75-76, 91-92
   health benefits of, 62, 69, 72-73, 103, 198, 239, 260-262
   motivation for, 30-31, 70-73, 76, 77
   stress-relief through, 71, 72, 123, 125

fainting, 62, 275
family history, 32, 42, 47, 49, 51-55, 65, 131-132, 135, 222, 233-234, 271-273
Famvir, 179
fast food, 17, 97, 257-258, 270

lipid profile, 14, 49-50, 159
liver disease, 18, 180
locker room, 22-23, 146
low-density lipoprotein (LDL), 49, 82, 83
  see also cholesterol
lung cancer, 17, 18, 20, 48, 54, 83, 261
lutein, 83
lycopene, 83, 221
lymph system, 45, 59, 225, 226, 228, 248

magnesium, 82
marijuana, 15, 198
massage, 126, 150
  prostatic, 240, 241
masturbation, 147, 170, 201, 202, 205
media images, 3, 25-26
medical history, 41, 42, 43, 64, 159, 234,
  271
  family, 32, 42, 47, 49, 51-55, 65, 131-
    132, 135, 222, 233-234, 271-273
medication, 14, 41-44, 64, 82, 109, 132-
  133, 178, 179, 256, 258-261, 271, 256
  side effects of, 107, 155, 157, 158, 159,
    162, 200-201, 210, 211, 231, 236-
    237, 249-250, 255
meditation, 126, 239
melanoma, 17, 57, 118
melatonin, 109, 210-211
menopause, 2, 209
men's groups, 3, 32-33, 70-71, 254-255
metabolism, 91, 92, 93, 209
Mexican food, 86, 96
midlife, 2-4, 69, 119, 209-215
minerals, 15, 81-84, 263
miscarriage, 182, 197-198
monogamy, 175, 184
morning-after pill, 191-192
mother-son relationship, 24, 35-36, 272
motorcycles, 16, 112-113
multiple sclerosis, 159
mumps, 200
muscle, 71, 73-77, 78, 90, 91, 92, 209,
  210, 211, 213, 231, 251
Muse, 166

nagging, 27, 73, 85, 95
nasal strips, 108
nausea, 262-264, 275
neck bruits, 45
neuropathy, diabetic, 158, 204, 261
nicotine patch, 105, 116
Novantrone, 233
numbness, 63, 158, 174, 258
nutrition, see diet

obesity, 49, 89, 108, 251, 253
older men, 34, 35, 71-72, 84, 89, 92, 152,
  212, 215
  sexual concerns of, 150-151, 152, 155,
    214
oral cancer, 17, 45, 115
oral tobacco, 15, 26, 36, 58, 115
organizations, medical, 72, 232-233, 242,
  283-284
osteoporosis, 35, 82, 213, 231

pain, 1-2, 23, 69, 72, 73, 130, 180, 230,
  233, 240, 252, 254, 256, 262, 274,
  275
paraphimosis, 250
Parkinson's disease, 132
Partin, Alan, 227
partner-exam, 55, 56, 57, 58-59, 154, 279
pasta, 79, 80, 86, 96-97
pelvic floor biofeedback, 164
penile cancer, 45, 56, 145, 178
penile implant, 156, 157, 160, 167-169, 174
penis size, 146-147
pets, 125
Peyronie's disease, 62, 147, 156, 160, 167,
  173-174, 203
phentolamine, 163
phimosis, 250
physical exam, 5, 14, 17, 30, 37-46, 51,
  65, 202-204, 220, 234-235, 260
  anxiety about, 42-43, 46, 47
  preparation for, 41-42, 234, 271
pneumonia, 18, 72
polyps, colon, 47, 54
potassium, 82
potatoes, 81, 82, 86, 97
pregnancy, 178, 180, 185, 190, 193, 207
priapism, 249-250
Prochaska, James, 27-28
Proscar, 231, 236
prostate, 16, 49, 104, 140, 147, 219-220
prostate cancer, 3-4, 18, 46, 48, 164, 211,
  212, 213, 219, 220-233, 261
  dietary factors in, 80-81, 83, 84, 221, 229
  family history of, 53, 54, 222
  research on, 19, 194, 219-220, 225,
    230, 232-233
prostate cancer screening, 14
prostate cancer support groups, 33
prostate enlargement, 140, 219, 223, 233-
  240, 256-258
prostate specific antigen (PSA) test, 49,
  53, 159, 213, 220, 222-223, 226, 227,
  229, 232, 235

About the Author

Ken Goldberg, M.D., is the founder and medical director of the Male Health Institute, the first center in the country specializing in health care for men. A board-certified urologist, Dr. Goldberg is the author of *How Men Can Live as Long as Women* and an adviser to *Prime Fitness* magazine, and his syndicated column "His Health" appears in newspapers across the country. He has been chosen as prostate educator for the south-central United States by the American Foundation for Urological Disease. For the past 10 years Dr. Goldberg has focused his interest on helping men live longer and better. He has treated and helped screen over 40,000 men. Dr. Goldberg lives in Dallas, Texas, with his wife, Sharon, and their two sons, Jeremy and Joshua.